MW00873852

Fix Your Fatty Liver

How I Naturally Reversed
And Healed My Fatty Liver

By Jonathan Mizel

Visit our website at: www.FixYourFattyLiver.com

First Printing: March 2018
ISBN 978-1985673267

Disclaimer and Terms of Use

Affiliate Referral Link Disclosure

GET YOUR FREE HEALTHY LIVER UPDATES, RECIPES, AND BONUSES BY REGISTERING HERE:

www.FattyLiverBook.com/fix

Introduction

Aloha, and welcome to the Fix Your Fatty Liver program!

My name is Jonathan Mizel and I created this program to share how I reversed and healed my fatty liver, and reclaimed my health. My goal is to help you do the same thing.

Up until the summer of 2014, my life was going along pretty good. Nice job, great family, wonderful friends. Overall, I felt very blessed. But you know what they say…

It's all for nothing if you don't have your health!

One beautiful Saturday morning, completely out of the blue, I woke up with a weird pain in my shoulder. I thought maybe I slept on it funny or pulled a muscle working in the yard.

I spent a whole month trying to ignore it, but it became harder and harder to brush aside, and there were numerous tell-tale signs something was wrong…

- I became unusually tired and didn't want to get out of bed. Normally I'm an early riser and a morning person.

- The whites of my eyes turned a light yellow and were often bloodshot. My skin became pale.

- I suddenly gained a bunch of extra weight I just couldn't get rid of. After meals, I felt bloated, like my food wasn't digesting. My whole body felt congested and fat.

- My eyesight got bad, and practically overnight, I had to buy stronger reading glasses.

- I became short-tempered and snapped at people I loved because I was in physical pain, and I didn't know what to do.

After a month, my wife looked at me said…

"You are going to the doctor… today!"

The appointment started out simple, a short drive to the clinic, some chit-chat with the nurse, a friendly catch-up with my doctor, then a blood test to check liver function (and *confirm* his suspicions). When the results finally came back, my life changed.

That's because a few days later, after more blood work and a very expensive CT scan (which wasn't covered by insurance), I was **officially** diagnosed with Fatty Liver Disease.

As you may know, fatty liver isn't a condition where you take a pill and it clears up in a few weeks. In fact, even though it affects almost **100 million people** in the US *alone*, there's no "official" cure.

Heck, there's not even a standard treatment plan!

That frustrated me, and it's when I began my quest…

- ✦ I resolved to learn how my body and liver functioned, and how to *naturally* support it instead of harming it with toxic food and a lifestyle that was obviously making me sick.

- ✦ I vowed to take responsibility for my health, instead of leaving it up to someone else.

- ✦ I promised myself I would help others who found themselves in the same boat, people with Nonalcoholic Fatty Liver Disease (NAFLD), Nonalcoholic Steatohepatitis (NASH), and Alcoholic Fatty Liver Disease (AFLD), and share what I discovered after I proved to myself it worked.

My goal is to give you the truth about how to change your life and heal your body. To transform the way you think about your liver, to shift your diet (and consciousness) and give you the hope and the tools to become healthy and happy again.

See, when the doctor gave me my diagnosis, I was shocked because…

- ✦ I didn't *think* I had a poor diet (I was wrong).

- ✦ I didn't *believe* I was purposely exposing myself to toxins (also wrong).

- ✦ And I certainly didn't *realize* how unhealthy or stressful my life had become (bordering on deadly).

There were plenty of times since my diagnosis when I felt like I might die…

…and more than a few times when I wanted to, because **I was in so much pain**. I'm not trying to be overdramatic, I just want you to know it was serious.

So I used my years of research skills and started a deep-dive on the topic of fatty liver, and lo and behold, I uncovered case after case where the patient was able to reverse their condition naturally, in most cases with dietary changes only.

I also did quite a bit of self-experimentation (known as Bio-Hacking) to find out what actually worked. And thankfully, after a long and painful journey, I climbed out of my hole, healed myself, and am back on my feet as far as my health is concerned.

My extra weight is gone, my body is strong, and I no longer suffer from a debilitating and compromised liver. In fact, my most recent blood tests show me at **completely normal** levels, and they have been that way for over a year now.

This program reveals what I did to reverse my liver problems, and how you **may** be able to do the same thing. I use the word **may** because I don't know you, I'm not a doctor, and I don't know what point you are starting from.

I will say that everything in this program is backed by the latest available science, or it has a long-term history of working. Chinese medicine and Ayurvedic practices are thousands of years old and have millions of followers (not to mention an established track-record of success).

Conventional medicine, while it has limitations, gives us access to modern test results, scientific research papers, physical data about our bodies, and exactly what's going on in there.

When you marry the two… magic happens!

Listen, every one of us are different people with different bodies. You'll want to try this for yourself to determine which parts have an impact on your liver and your health.

The best thing about this program is that you can go as deep as you like, based on how damaged your liver is, how much healing you need, and how open you are to the possibility of good health.

There really is no downside. The foundation of everything we recommend is rooted in basic 'good practices' for healthy living.

There Are 5 Pillars To Reversing Your Fatty Liver…

1 – **Proper Food and Nutrition**: For a majority of people reading this, a few simple dietary tweaks will start their recovery process. Food really is the most **important part** of healing your liver and fixing your life, which is why we cover what to eat and drink (and what **not** to eat and drink) in great detail.

As Hippocrates said in 431 B.C... "Let food be thy medicine and medicine be thy food." Think of what you eat as your first line of defense against disease and sickness. Fill your body with healthy delicious food instead of processed junk, and it will reward you with abundant health and a long, happy life.

2 – Non-Toxic Environment: There are all sorts of dangerous liver toxins you may be exposing yourself to, some without your knowledge. From medications to cleaning supplies to bug-spray. Heck, even your sunscreen may be poisoning your liver, and making you sick (I'll give you several alternatives later in this book).

In many cases, removing these chemical compounds from your life will start the healing and allow your liver to begin naturally rebuilding itself.

3 – Positive Mindset: There's scientific proof that breathing exercises and meditation can change your nervous system and help you dissolve stress, and specifically stress hormones. If you are nervous or agitated, that's probably harming your liver more than you realize.

We cover quite a few "positive attitude" secrets in this program. If you are new to that way of thinking, please give them a shot (you might be surprised). The affirmations and breathing exercises are a great way to start your day. Enjoy as many of these as you are comfortable with, and make them your own.

4 – Physical Movement: Erase the word *exercise* from your vocabulary and replace it with *movement*. Instead of "working out," take a walk in nature, a swim down at the local community center, a yoga class, or just a bike ride into town.

Learn how to stretch and breathe, something everybody needs, but almost nobody does. Maybe join a gym, or just go outside and move around.

5 – Supplements: Many people with fatty liver use vitamins and herbs to jumpstart the process. There are 13 specific supplements we cover in this program, which are the most recognized ones for liver issues.

Even if you aren't a "supplement" person, you might want to take a good probiotic every day and eat digestive enzymes with big meals. Vitamin C, E, turmeric, dandelion greens, and milk thistle can all help with a fatty liver.

But I want to get clear, food is the **most important** part of this program, and there is no magic pill that will solve all your problems. There are, however, some supplements that may aid in the healing process.

How Much Will It Cost To Implement This?

One of the things people ask is 'How much money do I need to budget to reverse my fatty liver?'

Since this is primarily a food-based program that's 100% natural (no pharmaceuticals or prescription drugs), it's not expensive to start. In fact, you might even spend less than you are currently spending on your "normal" unhealthy food!

Not to mention you'll save money on doctor visits, pain relievers, sleeping pills, and other over-the-counter medications, and actually **doing** something about your condition, as opposed to just treating the symptoms. Even the supplements we recommend are inexpensive, and in many cases, they are completely optional.

So to answer the question, we designed this program to be as affordable as possible, with a focus on **eating healthy food** and moving your body without personal trainers or expensive gym memberships.

Transform Your Body And Life!

Our hope is that you will take some (or all) of this info, and use it to reverse and heal your own fatty liver, to restore the good health you were born with, and to achieve the happiness you deserve.

And if it works for you, please send give us a testimonial so we can share this program with others, and impact their lives too.

Enjoy and have a blessed day,

Jonathan Mizel
Maui, Hawaii

Have Feedback Or A Testimonial? Share It Here:
FattyLiverBook.com/feedback

PART I: YOUR AMAZING LIVER

CHAPTER 1
All About Your Liver

The liver is one of the most important organs in the human body.

As one of the 5 vital organs, it is literally essential to your survival. Your liver helps more than 400 different bodily functions work properly, and it supports all your other organs, including your brain, heart, lungs, skin, and kidneys.

What exactly is an organ?

An organ is an integral part of a living organism with at least two different groups of tissues, and that performs at least one specific function. The human body contains 78 minor and major organs, spread across 12 organ systems.

These organ systems are responsible for the physical and mental processes that allow you to move and think. They influence your circulation, heart health, how you breathe, your immunity against infection and disease, your digestion and whether or not you can remember where you left your car keys.

Pretty much the whole kit and caboodle.

The liver works to support **all other organs** by keeping your blood pure and your body detoxified. It's crucial that it's strong and healthy. When your liver is happy, your overall health and well-being is too.

What Does The Liver Do?

First, let's consider the liver in a broad sense. It's **biggest** role is to separate the good from the bad. Some of what we consume is healthy, some of it isn't. The liver takes the healthy stuff and sends it into your body, where it's processed and used for nourishment. It takes the unhealthy stuff and prepares it to be eliminated through your bowels.

Now, I'm going to get a little science-y for a moment but stick with me, because by the end of Chapter 2, you'll know **exactly** why the liver is so important.

Every organ has at least 2 specific jobs. For the roughly 3 pound liver, the **main** function is filtering red blood cells from your blood, turning them into bile, passing them to your digestive tract, and then sending the filtered blood back into the body.

Your liver is holding, and processing, about 13% of your entire body's blood supply at any given time. That 1 pint of blood moves through 2 main lobes and thousands of lobules, at the rate of more than 2 quarts of blood per minute.

A full 25% of the blood pumped by your heart is processed by your liver. Additionally, all of the blood which leaves your intestines and your stomach passes through the liver too.

The enzymes produced by the liver mix with partially digested food, and aid in the removal of waste material. That's how you metabolize proteins, fats, and carbohydrates, the enzymes break them down, and help you absorb vitamins, minerals, and glycogen. Your liver even regulates whether or not your blood clots properly, and synthesizes certain plasma proteins.

In the process of purifying your blood, the liver removes chemicals and compounds that are poisonous or harmful to your body. It handles so many important functions necessary for human life that many doctors call it the "Grand Central Station" of your body.

But it would be wrong to say that the liver is primarily related to digestion. It also regulates blood sugar levels and metabolism, playing a major role in all of your metabolic processes, which is why a healthy liver helps you maintain a proper body weight.

In simple terms, the liver processes **anything** and **everything** you drink, eat, breathe or that gets absorbed into your skin, and either puts it to use in your body or helps eliminate it.

How Does The Liver Work?

We mentioned the main job of the liver is to filter and purify your blood. Oxygen-rich blood flows into your liver through the hepatic portal vein after it leaves your small intestine.

Blood from your portal vein may also contain toxic substances which were picked up through the skin and lungs. Once they hit the liver, it goes to work separating poisonous contaminants, and it begins processing them for removal.

It does that by releasing them to your colon to be eliminated. When it encounters healthy nutrients, fats, protein, and carbohydrates, it metabolizes them, storing them for later use, or releasing them back into your bloodstream.

For example, if you drink any type of alcohol, your liver is responsible for removing it from your blood. When you take medicine, your liver processes that medication, removing any unnecessary byproducts and tagging them for elimination, while retaining the health-boosting properties of the medication and sending it back into your blood flow or wherever it's needed.

When you eat food with carbohydrates or sugar, your liver senses this and reacts appropriately. To reduce glucose fluctuation in your body, your liver will pull that sugar from the blood, which comes in through the portal vein.

It stores this in the form of glycogen and releases it into the blood when sugar levels are too low. It also pulls vitamins and minerals like copper and iron out of incoming blood, releasing them when they are needed.

How All Your Organs Depend On The Liver

All the organs in your body rely on a healthy liver so they can function properly. For example, consider the skin.

The skin is your *largest* organ. It is the first layer of defense in your immune system. When you experience skin conditions, your liver is often to blame. An unhealthy liver may not be able to break down toxins and other poisons, so it sends them back through into your bloodstream, when they contaminate the skin from the "inside out."

This results in unsightly spots, eczema, dermatitis, rashes, psoriasis, acne, rosacea and other skin conditions … in large part because of an unhappy liver.

Many people go to the dermatologist for their skin problems, but in reality, they should probably try avoiding alcohol and foods that are known to damage the liver first. In cases where the liver is to blame, the key is not a cream or salve (which just treats the symptoms), but a shift in diet.

Liver And Heart Health

Fatty liver disease is also often associated with Metabolic Syndrome and coronary conditions that increase your risk of heart disease, stroke, high blood pressure, and heart attacks, often with very few symptoms.

People with nonalcoholic fatty liver disease (NAFLD) were found in one study to have higher instances of coronary artery disease than people without NAFLD. This makes sense when we go back to the liver's main job, acting as a filter.

When blood is not filtered properly due to liver disease, unhealthy blood literally **pollutes** your heart, keeping it from doing its main job of pumping clean, oxygenated blood throughout your body.

Your heart relies on a healthy liver in another way as well. One of the main jobs of the liver is to produce bile. Bile breaks down fat in your blood vessels. Your liver cranks out as many as 2 cups of bile each day. Why is bile so important?

Without it, fat stays in your blood and your arteries harden. This makes them smaller, restricting flow, increasing pressure, and resulting in your heart having to work harder than normal to circulate blood throughout your body.

When your heart has to work too hard for too long, you know what happens... a heart attack, stroke, or coronary thrombosis, which can kill you.

Liver And Brain Function

A buildup of toxins in the bloodstream because of an improperly functioning liver can also cause a decline in brain function and even brain damage. Your brain communicates with your body through the nervous system. Neurotransmitters send electrical messages that tell different parts of your body what to do and how to perform.

A brain weakened by toxic blood can release unhealthy levels of certain neurotransmitters and hormones, which means increased inflammation and stress throughout your body. Inflammation is at the foundation of many problematic and chronic diseases and illnesses.

The good news is that quite a bit of inflammation can be avoided with your diet, as we will look at shortly.

Digestion And Gallbladder Health

Literally, every part of your body, from head to toe, every major and minor organ, and all the body processes essential to human life, are impacted one way or the other by the health of your liver.

But the symptoms most often experienced in the early stages of liver disease are **digestive issues** and **excess fat storage**, especially in the belly, thighs, and love handles. Though all liver symptoms should be investigated, rapid weight gain (or even weight loss) is a big red flag that something is wrong. Let's look at how your liver is connected to your gallbladder,

Your gallbladder rests under the right lobe of your liver, which it relies on to produce bile. Bile is a digestive liquid that mixes with the food you eat, allowing it to be processed by your body. If your liver has done its job properly, there is plenty of bile in your gallbladder to help digest your food.

When you eat food containing fats, your gallbladder releases some of its stored bile, which breaks down the larger pieces of fat into smaller, more easily digestible components.

When your liver is healthy, you can effectively process dietary fat. But when it's sick, the fat you eat tends to stay in and around the liver, and in **extreme** cases, even leech into your body, contaminating your blood and altering your hormonal balance.

If you have been overweight and unable to lose excess pounds (especially in the belly, thighs, and love handles) it could be an unhealthy liver is at least partially to blame.

Beyond fat excretion, bile plays another very important role: It allows your body to absorb many vitamins and nutrients.

A healthy liver produces enough bile so that all the good components in the food you eat are absorbed into your body during digestion, while harmful and unneeded waste products are passed through and excreted when you go to the bathroom.

Can Your Liver Health Influence Your Hormones and Emotions?

Remember earlier when we talked about how an unhealthy liver negatively affects your brain? This is because toxins and hormones which are usually filtered out are still present, and they make it to your brain via blood flow, which causes inflammation.

Brain inflammation can make you feel "foggy" and "out of sorts," as well as irritable, tired, sluggish and depressed. *And* it can also affect your hormones.

One of the many things your liver regulates is hormonal balance. The liver is even known as the "Seat of Anger" in Traditional Chinese Medicine (TCM). When it does not filter hormones properly, the result is a hormonal imbalance. This imbalance may cause you to feel aggressive, overly reactive, and even angry for no reason.

Improper filtration in the liver can also lead to the overabundance of cortisol, appropriately referred to as "The Stress Hormone." Too much cortisol in your body means you feel extra physical and mental stress. This excess stress and anxiety drives your emotions, and not in a positive way.

Finally, cortisol also promotes excess weight gain, obesity and a host of medical problems related to being overweight. If you have struggled to lose weight using multiple diet plans and exercise programs, the issue might just be a fatty liver and its effect on cortisol and hormone production in addition to gallbladder function.

Simply put… keep your liver healthy and happy, and your hormones and emotions will be as well.

CHAPTER 2

What Is Fatty Liver?

According to the Mayo Clinic, as many as **100 million people** in the United States may have a fatty liver. That's more than 1 in 3 adults!

Appropriately called fatty liver disease, it occurs when excess fat builds up inside your liver cells, usually considered anything over 5%. This excess fat literally overwhelms it, replacing healthy tissue with fatty tissue.

Fatty liver is largely the result of unhealthy lifestyle choices, toxic environmental factors, and poor eating habits.

Unfortunately, fatty liver often doesn't produce symptoms until the condition has become a real health concern. You could have a fatty liver right now, which is creating a myriad of health problems, and not even know if you don't get tested.

Even if you do, it's often misdiagnosed. Many of the existing tests are not 100% accurate. Only ultrasound, CT scans, and MRIs can detect scarring, and only a biopsy can detect your liver's actual fat content and reveal damage.

These tests can be quite expensive and in the case of a biopsy, quite invasive. Undetected and untreated, more and more fat begins to take over healthy liver mass. This decreases the effectiveness of your metabolism and causes your body to burn fat less efficiently, which can morph into the inability to lose weight naturally.

Of course, this is not always the case. You can develop fatty liver without becoming overweight or obese, and some people actually lose weight, because their bodies start to break down from lack of nutrition.

Thankfully, your liver has an incredible ability to regenerate and renew itself, which means you should create a healthy environment for yourself, eat properly, and take other steps in this program to prevent the problem from worsening or happening in the first place.

The Different Types of Fatty Liver

The term fatty liver was first coined by the Mayo Clinic in 1980 as cases grew and doctors didn't know how to describe them. The most common type of liver disease in industrialized countries is called

Nonalcoholic Fatty Liver Disease (or NAFLD) and it's just one form of fatty liver. It refers to a condition that develops from causes not related to alcohol.

On the other hand, Alcoholic Fatty Liver Disease (AFLD) develops because of excessive alcohol consumption, to the point where it severely damages and scars the liver on a cellular level.

Let's take a look at the different stages of fatty liver, from benign to very serious.

Simple Fatty Liver Disease

All livers contain some fat, that's natural. But when that fat exceeds 5%, liver function starts to falter, and that's the point where doctors will make the diagnosis. Fat cells have taken over where liver cells normally exist, and the ability of the liver to do its job becomes limited.

Non-Alcoholic Fatty Liver Disease (NAFLD)

This is the most common condition. When the liver's fat content exceeds 5%, you are considered to be in a state of steatosis. This means fats and lipids are **stuck** inside the liver and are unable to be eliminated via normal function. It's estimated this condition affects as many as 1 in 3 people in the United States, and similar rates are seen in other modernized, first world nations like the UK, Australia, and Canada.

Because its symptoms mirror so many other common diseases and ailments, experts say this condition is drastically under-reported and misdiagnosed.

If you have some other health problem that hasn't been cleared up with traditional treatment methods, NAFLD could be the cause of your problem. There are *technically* two types of NAFLD: NAFL and NASH.

1. **NAFL**

A nonalcoholic fatty liver (NAFL) is when there is no inflammation due to the fat buildup. This is the most common cause of a liver disorder in the United States and other Western industrialized countries. The liver works normally and it even looks normal when cells are viewed under a microscope.

There could be a slight increase in your alanine transaminase (ALT) and aspartate transaminase (AST) liver enzymes. In most cases, simple NAFL can be reversed following the guidelines in this ebook, especially when it is caught early.

2. NASH

Nonalcoholic steatohepatitis (NASH) is when inflammation and the development of both fat and scar tissue are present in the liver. As opposed to NAFL, this means your liver enzyme levels are elevated above normal and are often accompanied by actual pain.

Because of heightened liver enzymes, inflammation, and scarring, a NASH diagnosis is more serious than having typical nonalcoholic fatty liver, and it can take longer to recover from. **This is what I was diagnosed with. It was very frightening at the time.**

Alcoholic fatty liver disease (AFLD)

If you are diagnosed with alcoholic fatty liver disease (AFLD), I have some really good news for you. Eliminating your alcohol intake is sometimes **all you need to do** to get your liver back on the road to normal functionality. Add a smart diet and regular physical movement and your liver becomes even healthier (and you also lose weight).

But if you continue to drink alcoholic beverages, even in moderation, you could develop alcoholic hepatitis or even worse, cirrhosis. Once cirrhosis occurs, abstinence cannot reverse the damage, and though it won't get any worse, your liver will forever be compromised.

However, complete abstinence can lessen the severity and prevent further damage from occurring. AFLD is more problematic than NAFLD because if left untreated, death can occur, so please pay attention if your doctor gives you a diagnosis of AFLD, and take a **complete break** from alcohol.

The Global Fatty Liver Phenomenon

Unfortunately, fatty liver disease has become quite common in the United States, and as I mentioned before, Europe, Australia, UK, India, and even China are all seeing increased cases.

Most of those countries have followed the US as far as dietary habits, eating what we have appropriately named S.A.D.

That acronym stands for the **Standard American Diet**, which means lots of processed foods: Simple carbohydrates, soda pop, refined sugars, white flour, meat and saturated fats, combined with eating little or no fresh vegetables, fruits, grains or other healthy plant-based foods.

In cultures where a plant-based diet is normal, instances of fatty liver, heart disease, neurological disorders, diabetes and other significant health problems have not reached an epidemic level like they have in places where S.A.D. is the norm.

It's not great that you got fatty liver, but it *is* great that this set into motion your own personal journey of improvement. Let this program be your first step in a long line of discoveries about how to live a full and happy life.

Pregnancy and Fatty Liver Disease

Be aware that pregnant women may build up fat in their liver as well, more than a normal and healthy amount. If you have fatty liver symptoms, before or during your pregnancy, make sure your OBGYN or doctor knows that, and monitors both you and your baby.

This only happens in extremely rare cases, but risks exist for both the pregnant mom-to-be, as well as the unborn child. Kidney failure is sometimes a possibility, as well as increased bleeding.

Doctors don't fully understand what causes a fatty liver during pregnancy, though they believe hormones are a key factor. If you are diagnosed with fatty liver during pregnancy, follow your doctor's instructions carefully. You want to avoid increasing the chance that fatty liver and the accompanying health risks could transfer to your child.

It is important to note that most fatty liver diseases and conditions, regardless of which type you have, are treatable. Behavioral, dietary and environmental changes are usually all that is needed to prevent, and even reverse liver problems, which cause many other physical and mental health issues as well.

CHAPTER 3

Why Are Fatty Liver Cases Growing?

After reading about the main causes of fatty liver, you may feel overwhelmed.

You might be looking around your environment right now, whether you are at work, at home, or at play, wondering *exactly* what influences are raising your risk for developing or worsening this dangerous condition.

If you are scolding yourself for not exercising more or eating things you know you shouldn't, that's understandable.

However, be aware there are forces at work, **dark forces** say some, and you are not completely to blame for many of the health problems you have. This is because food manufacturers, as well as politicians and others who play a key role in telling you what you should be eating, have been giving you the **wrong information** for decades, and it appears they've been doing so intentionally.

This isn't meant to sound like some sort of unfounded conspiracy theory.

The way modern humans have become so sick, fat and unhealthy is a matter of public record. Big agricultural companies, especially wheat and meat farmers, sugar manufacturers, and others with billions at stake in multiple agricultural industries, have paid health authorities to recommend their products, even when they know they are making you sick, and in some cases killing you.

We also saw this in the massive lawsuits brought against the tobacco industry. The Tobacco Master Settlement Agreement (MSA) was the result of lawsuits in the US started by the Attorneys General of 46 states. They sued the Big 4 tobacco companies for recovery of tobacco-related health care costs and made certain practices illegal.

As a result of this massive lawsuit, more people were made aware of the deadly effects of smoking. As CNN reported in November of 2015, smoking has been on an impressive decline ever since that lawsuit.

Even so, the legal action goes to show one important point about the pursuit of money in relation to product manufacturers' level of concern about your health and well-being…

When the money gets big enough, companies will do whatever it takes to misinform and downright lie to keep you buying their products, even if your health and very existence are threatened.

This is what has led to the proliferation of the S.A.D. eating habits of modern human beings. **Food manufacturers strip nutrition from healthy, natural foods.** The simple reason why is because then those products will last longer on grocery store shelves.

When they pull nutrition out of healthy plant-based foods, what do they replace it with? Refined sugars, simple carbohydrates, unhealthy fats, extremely high levels of salt, preservatives and chemicals all meant to do just 3 things:

1 – Give the product a longer shelf life.

2 – Keep manufacturing costs down by using inexpensive additives and ingredients to bulk up weight and volume of food.

3 – Create a pleasurable response in your brain that often leads to an addiction some say is *more powerful* than cocaine.

It's a failure of society when poor quality food is addictive and harmful to the human body, and even worse when it's the only option available. In the United States, the UK, Canada and other modernized nations, there are vast wastelands of nutrition known as "food deserts."

That term refers to populated areas where healthy food like fresh fruits and vegetables are more than 1 mile away from most residents.

In those same areas, there are dozens of fast food restaurants and small, corner stores that sell predominantly processed and refined foods, alcohol, soda pop, candy, chips, and other junk that's directly harming the people who live there.

When fresh vegetables and fruits are nearby, they are often out of the financial reach of the residents of food deserts, who can easily walk to a fast-food joint right down the street for some cheap, addictive and unhealthy fast food.

You may find yourself from time to time eating food that is less than healthy. We all do it, because it's convenient, inexpensive, and literally staring you in the face everywhere you go. Just remember this type of eating is likely why you have fatty liver. Go for an apple or orange instead.

The History of the Modern-Day Food Pyramid

How many fast food and casual dining restaurants do you see on a daily basis, as opposed to fresh vegetable and fruit stands? We have arrived at the sad state in our evolution where it's easier to get unhealthy processed junk over health boosting plant-based foods, and a big reason is the Modern-Day Food Pyramid.

We look to our political leaders to protect us. We vote for people we hope are going to look out for our best interests. Unfortunately, these leaders often wind up doing just the opposite.

Let's look at little timeline:

1917 - The first US food guide appeared in the United States. Caroline Hunt, a nutritionist working for the USDA (United States Department of Agriculture) advised limiting fat and sugar intake while recommending getting more vegetables and minerals into the body. Not a bad start.

1956 - This evolved into the Basic 4 food groups, namely milk, meat, fruits/vegetables, and grain products. This made a square, and it's where the term "square" meal came from because it was substantial and satisfying, even though it was heavy on meat and dairy.

1967 - Senator George McGovern formed and headed the Select Committee on Nutrition and Human Needs, establishing dietary guidelines based on real science.

1977 - The Select Committee on Nutrition and Human Needs told Americans to cut back on saturated fat and cholesterol consumption by as much as 60%. The recommendations proposed reducing your meat and dairy intake in the name of better health.

And this is where things start to go downhill...

You see, the egg, cattle and dairy industries were not too happy with this because consumption of their core products began to fall. It wasn't long before these manufacturers decided to influence what Americans were told to eat. They would not stand idly by and watch their industries suffer, even if factual information proved their products as less than healthy.

This was the beginning of the USDA food pyramid, which recommends eating large daily quantities of food at its base, tapering down to little or none of the food at the pyramid's point.

1980 - When the first US food pyramid appeared, it was **highly** influenced by big money across the agriculture industry, and in many cases, it ignored proven nutrition links to good and bad health.

A woman named Luise Light worked for the USDA at the time the pyramid was originally developed. She was one of a group of top nutritionists tasked with creating the first model.

She stated in numerous interviews that the original food pyramid for the United States was *"...sold to the highest bidder."* The following is a direct quote:

"When our version of the Food Guide came back to us, we were shocked to find that it was vastly different from the one we had developed. As I later discovered, the wholesale changes made to the guide by the Office of the Secretary of Agriculture were calculated to win the acceptance of the food industry.

For instance, the AG Secretary's office altered wording to emphasize processed foods over fresh and whole foods, to downplay lean meats and low-fat dairy choices because the meat and milk lobbies believed it would hurt sales of full-fat products; it also hugely increased the servings of processed wheat and other grains to make the growers happy.

The meat lobby got the final word on the color of the saturated fat/cholesterol guideline, which was changed from red to purple because meat producers worried that using red to signify "bad" fat would be linked to red meat in consumers' minds."

Light and her nutritionist colleagues recommended 3 to 4 daily servings of whole grains, bread and cereals. The wheat and corn industries paid the right politicians enough money to get that changed to 6 to 11 servings per day, and include highly processed grains that were far less healthy, but had a long shelf life and could be adulterated with sugar, fat, and sodium.

The **science** said to eat little or no baked goods, crackers, sweets or other *"low-nutrient foods laden with sugars and fats."* Yet, those ended up as the **base** of the pyramid and became the foundation, rather than something to be eaten sparingly.

The nutritionists also recommended specific wording to *"eat less"* processed foods, junk foods, and fast foods. As a nod to the manufacturers of these unhealthy and addictive foods, that wording was changed to *"avoid too much"* of those products.

The definition of "too much" was never given.

The United States is far from the only country that has government organizations recommending unhealthy food habits. It turns out politicians in other countries have their pockets lined with money from interested food manufacturers, too.

The largest food processors and agricultural companies have a global presence, which is why their less-than-healthy foods cause a **worldwide** epidemic of overeating, diabetes, obesity, and in turn, high rates of fatty liver. Often with very little repercussions, and billions of dollars at stake, these companies have few limits on their influence.

The Sugar/Fat War May be Responsible For Your Fatty Liver

The unhealthy, and much too common, Standard American Diet referenced throughout this program had its beginnings in the 1960s. Documents obtained by the Journal of the American Medical Association (JAMA) show that the sugar industry blatantly funded research to incorrectly and intentionally downplay the health risks while pointing to fat as the cause of many health problems.

The truth is though, that both fat **and** sugar are to blame for many of the health issues we have today. Internal documents taken from sugar industry companies show that sugar manufacturers have largely influenced today's dietary recommendations, intentionally lying about the link between sugar and heart disease.

In 1967, the sugar industry paid today's equivalent of $50,000 to 3 Harvard researchers to compile research on fat, sugar, and their links to heart disease.

Big Sugar cherry-picked studies from their paid researchers. They then released watered-down findings, minimizing the very real link between sugar and heart disease, making fat out to be the villain.

Recent documentation shows more of the same unethical behavior. Major soft-drink manufacturers have paid millions to show that sugary drinks such as theirs have no link to obesity, even though that's not true.

The Associated Press in September of 2016 reported candy manufacturers are working to prove that kids who eat candy, devoid of all nutrition, actually weigh less than those who don't eat sugary sweets.

Why is this happening? Simple…

They Want To Make You Addicted To Their Products

Drug dealers don't talk about the dangerous effects of their products. Instead, they remind you of how good their products make you feel, maybe even give you a free sample to get you hooked.

Make no mistake about it... sugar and processed food manufacturers are even **more of a threat** to your health than a drug dealer because they are allowed to legally advertise on TV and the Internet.

Like a drug dealer, they regularly tell you (and your kids), how yummy their products are, while ignoring the actual health risks. These companies have been shown to misinform the public about how their products are killing people, and it seems like they just don't care. (Lightbulb moment: they don't!)

The fact is, you eat food 3 - 5 times a day, and most people will simply choose what's convenient, available, and affordable over what's healthy.

They know this, and want you and your children eating **their** foods and drinking **their** sodas, rather than fresh natural foods they can't profit from. That is why they spend billions on advertising, and who-knows-how-much lining the pockets of greedy politicians and others who are in charge of telling you what is and is not healthy to eat.

Don't get me wrong, I believe in open markets, and customer options, and freedom of choice. But the level of **deception and manipulation** in the food industry means that our choices are anything but free.

40 Sneaky Ways Food Manufacturers "Hide" Sugar

While we're on the topic of sugar, let's take a closer look at that sweet toxin. Sugar is not necessarily a bad thing. There is sugar in fruits and even some vegetables, but that's not the problem.

It's when you consume an **overabundance in processed form** that your body suffers. Sugar consumption directly leads to fatty liver, diabetes, metabolic syndrome, and a host of other health issues. There's a great article on **exactly** what happens in your body when you load up on sugar in the resources at the back of this book.

The biggest problem is that people get way too much. The American Heart Association recommends no more than 100 calories (25 grams or 6 teaspoons) of *added* sugar **per day** for women. Men can probably get away with up to 150 calories (37.5 grams or 9 teaspoons) **per day**.

Be forewarned though, those are **maximums** that apply **only** to people with healthy livers. You want to dramatically reduce the amount of sugar you put into your body to speed up your recovery, and if possible, eat *no sugar* or foods containing added sugar during your healing process (plan for 60 - 90 days).

Now you may be looking at those numbers and thinking, "I don't use anywhere near that much added sugar!" The problem is that food manufacturers hide the sugar in processed food, and don't tell you about it.

This practice led to the average US resident consuming 306 calories of sugar each day in 2008, the equivalent of a whopping 77 grams or 19 teaspoons. According to the US Department of Agriculture, in 2016 daily consumption is up to 358 calories, that's 94 grams or **23 teaspoons**!

That means if you are an average person, you eat **three and a half times** too much sugar for women, **two times** too much for men.

As if adding unhealthy amounts of sugar to your food without asking first is not bad enough, the manufacturers figured out how to intentionally mislead you.

They list sugar as sugar, but also as the following 40 ingredients. Read your food labels. If any of the following items are present, you are looking at sugar. You will notice that in some cases there are multiple "sugar" ingredients on a single food label.

1 – High Fructose Corn Syrup	21 – Fruit Juice Concentrate
2 – Sucrose	22 – Malt Syrup
3 – Glucose	23 – Panocha
4 – Fructose	24 – Turbinado Sugar
5 – Lactose	25 – Syrup
6 – Maltose	26 – Muscovado Sugar
7 – Dextrose	27 – Raisin Syrup
8 – Honey	28 – Barbados Sugar
9 – Corn Syrup	29 – Sorghum Syrup
10 – Invert Sugar	30 – Refiner's Syrup
11 – Florida crystals	31 – Beet Sugar
12 – Molasses	32 – Carob Syrup
13 – Brown Sugar	33 – Table Sugar
14 – Evaporated Cane Juice	34 – Malt
15 – Sugar Crystals	35 – Buttered Syrup
16 – Treacle	36 – Maple Syrup
17 – Demerara Sugar	37 – Rice Syrup
18 – Fruit Juice Crystals	38 – Agave Nectar or Syrup
19 – Dehydrated Fruit Juice	39 – Powdered Sugar
20 – Corn Sweetener	40 – Confectioner's Sugar

Just remember that any food ingredient ending in "ose" is sugar, which means there are actually even more than 40.

Your body really doesn't need added sugar. In fact, it's been an evolutionary challenge for us it to handle it. Processed, refined sugar has zero nutritional value.

Contrast that with the sugar contained in fruits and vegetables, which is accompanied by fiber, water and healthy nutrients like vitamins and minerals. This volume helps make us feel full, and is one of the many reasons that, as long as you eat it in its natural form (and not in juice or treats), the sugars in fruits and vegetables are fine.

Naturally occurring sugar may have calories, but they aren't "empty" calories. And of course, they certainly are not poisonous like the refined stuff.

Food manufacturers know people are more aware of what they are putting into their bodies today than ever before. They understand that the average person is on the lookout for sugar in the foods they eat, and the beverages they drink.

So they choose **healthier** sounding names to try and pull the wool over our eyes and to keep fueling our addiction so we continue to buy their products.

Here are a few you might be familiar with, which you may **not** know contain as much added sugar as they do…

- A single cup of supposedly healthy low-fat fruit-flavored yogurt packs up to 47 grams or 200 calories of sugar. That's 12 teaspoons folks, a literal sugar-bomb, and nearly 50% *more* than what's in a can of soda. Much better to have a piece of fruit in the morning, like an apple, which gives you energy, fiber, and has zero refined sugar.

- A 20-ounce bottle of an average sports drink literally shocks your liver with 32 grams of sugar (159 calories, 8 teaspoons). Try water, or lemon water, or a green drink if you want some extra flavor. If you need something sweet, make a smoothie.

- Granola is often considered a "health" food, but it's usually loaded with sugar. A 100-gram serving delivers 6 teaspoons (23.5 grams, 100 calories). That can make you crash mid-morning. Oatmeal is a better option because it breaks down far slower, and delivers energy over 3 - 4 hours, vs. 1 hour for sweetened cereal.

- Many protein bars are no better than candy bars, at least as far as sugar content is concerned. There are dozens of protein bars that are packed with 30+ grams of added sugar (7.3 teaspoons, 149 calories). Better to have some nuts or dried fruit, and give yourself a boost instead of a crash.

- Even salty snacks often contain sugar. For example, a small frozen pizza contains 16 grams of sugar (or 3.2 teaspoons, 80 calories). Factor in the carbs, fats, sodium, and low-quality meat, and you literally have a recipe for giving yourself fatty liver disease.

- And even though you already know it's not good for you, it's worth noting the whopping sugar content in soda. A 12 ounce can of cola contains 140 calories of sugar (8.4 teaspoons, 33 grams). A good alternative is tea. Ice tea is just as refreshing and contains zero grams of sugar.

You may have thought some of those foods were healthy and safe, but if you have liver issues, they're not. That's why it is so important to **read food labels** and know what names manufacturers hide sugar under because honestly, they stick it in **everything** these days.

Since we're on the topic, let's talk about…

How To Properly Read Food Labels

Food manufacturers in the United States, the UK, and most other industrialized nations are required to list certain things on food labels. The number of servings, nutritional content, and daily recommended allowances are all things you will see on a food label.

But how can you make sense of all this information? It's actually quite simple when you use the following 4 step process…

1. Before you do anything else, **check the serving size.** All information on a food label pertains to a single serving, and many cans and packages contain more than 1 serving. The biggest scam is making a serving size much smaller than you what you actually end up eating!

2. Look at the ingredients listed with **measurements**, closer to the top and middle of the nutrition label. These are things like fat, cholesterol, sodium, carbohydrates, and protein. If you see 15g of sugar, that means 15 grams per serving, not per container. Do this with all of the ingredients listed, so you understand what impact you are having on the daily recommended allowances of healthy (and not so healthy) ingredients.

3. Then simply **do a little math**. Let's say a small slice of frozen apple pie lists the sugar content at 19 grams. However, because there are 8 servings in the package, and most people have *way more* than a small slice, that would be over your daily maximum, not counting everything else you eat that day.

4. Finally, look below the nutrition facts, figures, measurements, and daily value percentages. There is an area that says INGREDIENTS and then lists multiple items. Ingredients are always listed in descending order, from the most to the least weight and presence in the container. The foods listed first on the ingredients list are present in greater volume than those listed later.

Unfortunately, as of 2017 manufacturers were not required to list sugar as a percentage of a recommended daily allowance. There are several pieces of legislation in the United States pushing to change this.

You need to monitor and protect your own health. No one cares as much about your health and well-being as you do.

So if you ate the whole pie in the example above, you would have consumed **almost 700%** of the recommended daily allowance of added sugar for a woman, and **over 500%** for a man. From one lousy pie!

For ingredients other than sugar, like total fat, saturated fat, cholesterol, and sodium, you will receive both a measurement, usually in grams (g) or milligrams (mg), and a percent daily value figure on a food label.

Multiply your percent daily value times the number of servings on the food label. If there are 8 servings in a particular container, multiplying 8 servings x 12% of the daily recommended value of total fat per serving shows that the entire container delivers 96% of the total fat you should eat in one day. Once you get going, you'll find that the labels on your food can be quite shocking.

You Are Responsible For Your Health And Diet

You and you alone are your best health advocate. This is great news. It means that you can achieve super health and vitality when you get informed and uncover the truth.

Do your research. See what works for you. Pay attention to how certain foods make you feel after you eat them. Consult your doctor of course, but understand that when it comes to nutrition, many of them are ill-informed as well. The average doctor receives less that 20 hours of nutrition training, and that's over an 4 year period.

A professional nutritionist is often a better option, especially if they are trained in how specific foods combat disease.

When in doubt, eat more plant-based foods, choose organic whenever possible, and cook for yourself so you know what's in your food. Move around during the day. Take the stairs, walk to work, park further away. Drink lots of water and liquids.

Get plenty of rest, limit your environmental exposure to toxins and poisons, and realize that food manufacturers and your government are **not** who you should turn to for nutrition or health advice. You'll live a longer, happier life, free of a fatty liver and other major health problems.

In a perfect world, your doctor will forget about your fatty liver because you won't have it anymore, and your healthy living efforts will begin to pay off in overall wellness and happiness.

Oh yeah … and your liver will LOVE you!

Resources We Recommend

Over the past few years, there have been some great movies released on nutrition and the food business, and how those two things are often at odds with one another. Most of these are on Netflix or Amazon, and all are quite good.

If you are looking to take control over your diet, cure your fatty liver, get off medications, lose some weight, end your diabetes, or simply to live a healthier life, all of these will empower you by helping you to understand the forces that care more about their profit than your health.

- Forks over Knives
- Fed Up
- What the Health
- Fat, Sick, and Nearly Dead (Parts I and II)
- Food Matters
- Supersize Me
- Food Choices
- King Corn
- Food Inc.
- Hungry for Change
- Food Fight
- Our Daily Bread
- Plant Pure Nation

CHAPTER 4

Getting Your Diagnosis

Many people begin feeling tired and sluggish, seemingly, for no reason. They start to find it difficult to lose weight, even if they exercise. They feel a cramping in their belly, a soreness in their right side, their urine may become dark or brown, and their judgment gets sketchy since they have problems concentrating.

If you have two or more of these indicators, you need to consider fat buildup in your liver as a likely culprit, especially if you also have high blood pressure, high cholesterol, or diabetes.

Unfortunately, fatty liver may not become symptomatic right away. Years or even decades may pass before your liver fat content becomes high enough that health problems arise.

That's why it's so important to act **before** it becomes a serious threat. If your liver currently has too much fat, but you don't display classic symptoms, smart nutrition and other good health habits can **reverse** your condition before it manifests into something far more serious.

So, what are some symptoms that could indicate a fatty liver and have you headed to the doctor?

- Tiredness, sluggishness or fatigue
- Belly fat or extra weight in thighs, hips or live handles
- Patchy, dark areas on chest and back
- Red patches on neck skin and underarms
- Insulin resistance, pre-diabetes
- Pain in the upper right area of your stomach
- Soreness in back or right shoulder
- Yellow eyes and jaundiced skin
- Difficulty consuming alcohol
- High cholesterol levels
- Metabolic syndrome
- Heart disease
- Abdominal cramping
- Dark or brown urine
- Confusion, poor judgment, trouble concentrating
- Feeling weak and lifeless
- Nausea and digestive issues
- Some people even lose weight

A lot of fatty liver symptoms initially look like something else. That sore back could be caused from working in the garden. Nausea and abdominal pain could be from food poisoning or a gastrointestinal issue.

In both of those cases, you might believe time will heal you. But if you do indeed have fatty liver, ignoring your symptoms is *always* the worst course of action, because the worse it gets, the more likely the damage becomes permanent.

So, When Should You Consult a Doctor?

You have probably already seen a doctor, which is why you bought this program to begin with. But if you haven't, you shouldn't waste any time. If you display multiple symptoms and/or if they **get worse** and more numerous over time, see your doctor immediately.

A simple blood test will reveal abnormally high ALT and ALS enzymes that indicate an unhealthy liver. Doctors typically take blood samples from patients complaining of just about any condition, because it's a very good way to see exactly what is going on inside your body, plus a blood test can catch other things too.

In some cases, your doctor may also request an ultrasound, CAT scan, or MRI to get a clearer picture of your liver. As we mentioned, in extreme situations, a biopsy may take place. This is where a small part of your liver is removed. That liver sample is then observed under a microscope for signs of inflammation, damaged or dead liver cells and excess fat.

Even if your symptoms are mild, you should schedule an appointment with your doctor and get your blood tested to make sure you know what's happening in your body. If you don't have fatty liver disease, you could have some other condition, and no matter what is going on, you'll want to know what it is so you can take care of it before it gets worse.

Complications of Fatty Liver

You should always consult a trained medical professional when you display any indicators of poor health. This is especially true when you are showing signs of fatty liver disease.

If you keep putting off seeing your doctor, more serious health problems can arise down the line, which is what happened to me. These complications include, but are not limited to, the following:

- Obesity
- Type II diabetes
- High cholesterol
- Sleep apnea
- Coronary issues

- Gastrointestinal bleeding
- Cirrhosis of the liver
- Liver cancer
- Total liver failure

Remember, simple fatty liver disease is almost always treatable. Your liver is incredibly good at staying healthy. This is why symptoms don't appear for years in most cases. Your liver is actively fighting the fat buildup.

Over time though, when a poor diet, low levels of physical activity, or environmental issues continue to aggravate you, fatty liver begins to show physical symptoms.

How Long Does It Take To Reverse A Fatty Liver?

One question many people ask is how long does it take to reverse and heal a fatty liver? Days, weeks, months?

The truth is that fatty liver is often caused by many years of poor diet and living in a toxic, stressed-out, chemical-filled environment. Obviously, if that's the case, you aren't going to undo your damage overnight.

There are basically four grades of fatty liver:

Grade 1: Otherwise known as simple or Non-alcoholic fatty liver disease (NAFLD), this is what most people are diagnosed with. Grade 1 is where excess fat builds up within your liver cells, usually around 5% by weight. The good news is that NAFLD is almost always reversible.

Grade 2: Approximately 10% of all fatty liver cases progress to this level. It's medically referred to as Nonalcoholic Steatohepatitis (NASH). If you are at Grade 2, it means there is already some scarring of your liver. The good news is that NASH is often reversible, but because of the scarring, your liver may never return to 100% functionality. That means you need to be very careful about what you eat, drink, and any toxins you are exposed to.

Grade 3: Over time, if left untreated, your fatty liver will eventually progress to Grade 3, which indicates serious issues, including low functionality, cirrhosis, or fibrosis. At this point, you probably have multiple symptoms, including jaundice, abdominal pain, poor vision, weakness, and inflammation.

Grade 4: This is the point where the liver is beyond repair, and you may even need a liver transplant. Of course there are people who come back from this with good diet and a healthy lifestyle, but those cases are rare. Grade 4 is generally considered catastrophic since transplants are dangerous, expensive, and the long-term survival rate is quite low.

What's The Recovery Time?

The recovery time is based on your level of damage, and how willing you are to abstain from alcohol, sugar, and processed foods while you are healing.

The times below should be considered minimums…

- Recovery time for Grade 1: 3 – 6 months
- Recovery time for Grade 2: 6 – 12 months
- Recovery time for Grade 3: 1 – 2 years
- Recovery time for Grade 4: 2 – 3 years, possible liver transplant

Of course, if you continue to damage your liver with poor lifestyle habits, you may never fully recover. Your liver can rebuild itself, but you need to do your part.

Making conscious changes in your life now can prevent a health crisis from happening, and reverse this condition if it has already begun to develop.

CHAPTER 5

Assembling Your Healthy Living Team

Whenever you suffer from some serious sickness, disease or ailment, you should always consult a licensed physician or healthcare specialist. They have experience, training, and many tools at their disposal to help determine the extent of the damage, and what it might be caused from.

Rather than relying on just one person, I recommend you build a *team* of people, a support network who can help you analyze, investigate, and ultimately repair what's wrong with you, no matter what that is.

First on the list would be your General Practitioner, family doctor, hepatologist, or nutritionist. I put these people in the "conventional" category. They went to school, and while that doesn't mean they are miracle workers, it does indicate they are at least reasonably intelligent, and they've been professionally trained.

Your conventional health care providers will order and help you evaluate your test results, give you general advice, and should be seen as an essential part of the journey to reversing your condition.

Should You Also Turn to Alternative Medicine?

There are quite a few alternative practitioners these days, and I recommend you work with someone from that side of the fence too since they tend to be more attuned to liver issues, and also integrate things like mindset, meditation, herbs, acupuncture, nutrition, and when appropriate, supplements…

- Naturopathy is a medical system that evolved from traditional practices and European practices. Naturopaths go to school, and get a degree, a bit less rigorous than MDs, but are still well educated and able to diagnose and treat fatty-liver.

- Traditional Chinese Medicine (TCM) practitioners are often traditionally schooled. They practice a style of ancient medicine from China, though the best practitioners combine that knowledge with modern medicine, they also integrate herbal medicine, massage, movement, Ayurvedic practices and dietary therapy.

- Osteopathy is a type of alternative medicine that emphasizes massage and other physical manipulation of muscle tissue and bones.

- Chiropractic is a form of alternative medicine mostly concerned with the diagnosis and treatment of mechanical disorders of the musculoskeletal system, especially the spine. If you have joint pain, they may be able to help.

So in addition to your conventional doctor, I recommend you also have an alternative practitioner who can help you in times when your MD can't (or won't). I would stick with a naturopath or TCM doctor, but based on where you live and the availability in your area, you may have to be flexible.

Conventional medicine has become more and more aware in recent years of the power and validity of alternative therapies. This doesn't mean anyone who expresses knowledge should be brought on board your team, however.

You would not let a doctor operate on you if he told you he received his education by reading medical journals in his spare time. You would insist they went to the relevant schools, earned an accredited degree, and have actual experience treating what ails you.

Your medical doctor provides the modern-day treatments, tests, and medicines based on scientific research. Your alternative practitioner brings in established dietary practices, practical education, as well as supplements that may be able to help you heal.

Both of these dedicated health professionals together can help you positively approach, and reverse your fatty liver condition.

Get a buddy on board

Don't try to do this alone. Explain what is going on to your spouse, friend, co-worker, or whoever you have in your life that you can count on. It's nothing to be ashamed of, and extremely common these days. Having someone you are close to, that you can discuss your plan and options with, is generally a good idea for any big changes you are making in life.

It's possible the improvements you are going to make will have a positive effect on your buddy too, especially if they are a close friend or family member!

CHAPTER 6

How Did You Get Fatty Liver?

Okay, you have been diagnosed with a fatty liver. Your enzymes are out of whack, your liver is inflamed, and you have other symptoms too.

Unless time travel becomes possible, you have to stop worrying about the past. You cannot change the decisions you made yesterday, last year, or 10 years ago.

Beating yourself up mentally over why you ended up in this situation does no good. As a matter of fact, stressing out can actually make the matter worse, and cause your liver even more harm.

There are a couple of reasons for this…

First off, mental stress often causes people to reach for their favorite comfort foods. There is a reason they are called that. We find **comfort** in them. They make us feel good because of the crap manufacturers put in there, things like sugar, salt, fat, and monosodium glutamate (MSG), which cause an addictive reaction in your brain.

This triggers the release of dopamine, serotonin and other natural chemicals inside your body, which are known as "happy hormones." When we eat these incredibly unhealthy, nutrient-poor and addictive foods, they make us feel good for a **short period of time**, so we reach for them again and again to fight stress, anxiety, and depression.

And this stimulus-response makes us eat the exact foods that are killing us, and actually *want them more* than healthy foods.

Second reason why you should give up stress?

Worry and anxiety can effect you physiologically. They make you slouch, and keep you from sitting and standing up straight, which can stifle your blood flow. And they also effect your breathing, which means your liver is probably not getting enough oxygen, another reason it may be having trouble healing itself.

So, as long as you're headed in a positive direction, there's no need to beat yourself up about the past.

Why did you get it?

What you eat is the **main reason** for the development of fat in your liver. Changing those habits is the easiest way to reverse those conditions. There are a number of reasons why people develop fatty liver. We will list the common ones shortly, but a great deal of it has to do with toxic food and lack of nutrition.

Remember, most people have some fat in their liver. This is a natural phenomenon. Until it reaches 5% or greater, this fat is usually not an issue. But if you continue to eat junk rather than vegetables, fruits, or other high-fiber foods, you only make the problem worse.

How Obesity, Diabetes, and Fatty Liver Are Interrelated

The National Health Service in the United Kingdom, the National Institutes of Health in the United States, the Canadian Liver Foundation and countless health organizations around the world agree that the leading cause of fatty liver is obesity and diabetes.

The two go hand in hand: The more overweight you are, the higher your risk of fat infiltrating and "taking over" your liver. The more fat that ends up in your liver, the more difficult it is for your body to process new fats and sugars, and separate healthy food from the junk you consume.

- Health authorities in Canada estimate that more than 50% of Canadians are overweight or obese.

- In the United States, being heavy is even more of a problem, with every 2 out of 3 adults qualifying as overweight or obese.

- In the United Kingdom, a full 64% of adults earn the title of either overweight or obese.

- From 1980 to today, there has been a 55% increase in the number of people who became overweight or obese across the globe.

You probably don't need me to tell you that the reason for the weight problem epidemic in modern countries is the **quality of food** that the average person puts into his or her body.

The Standard American Diet was highlighted earlier as the typical eating practice of men, women, and children today. If you are old enough to remember, think back to the 1970s. Compare the number of fast food and processed food chain restaurants and casual dining destinations both then and now.

I remember when a famous fast food joint opened a few miles from my house in 1975. Back then it was considered a special treat, a place we would visit once a month, certainly not something to be consumed on a daily or even weekly basis.

There is a very good reason the increase in fatty liver, heart disease, obesity, diabetes, and cancer has grown in direct correlation with unhealthy food manufacturing processes and the stripping of nutrition from food…

What they serve isn't food at all, it's poison!

The term fatty liver was introduced by the Mayo Clinic in 1980. By then, the United States and other first world countries had been consuming more and more processed and fast foods on a regular basis, for about 5 to 10 years.

Child onset diabetes basically **did not even exist** before modern food manufacturing came to be, and now as many as 1 in 3 children born after the year 2000 will contract early onset diabetes.

Heart disease, cancer, and obesity have increased alongside "modern" food manufacturing practices, which strip nutrition from the food you eat and pump it full of preservatives, chemicals and compounds known to cause addiction and health problems.

Simply put, what you are eating can either make you healthy… or extremely unhealthy, with most people on this planet falling on the unhealthy side.

The stunning fact is, the main cause is well known… It's consuming a diet lacking in nutrition and plant-based foods, while also high in processed foods, refined sugars and simple carbohydrates. That, in a nutshell is how you give yourself fatty liver.

Additional Factors

In addition to diet, the following conditions, lifestyle behaviors, and influences are all known to significantly raise your risk of developing unhealthy levels of fat in your liver:

- Lack of regular physical activity
- Environmental influences and toxins
- Some medications
- Recreational drugs such as alcohol and tobacco
- A family history of liver disease or diabetes
- Being diabetic

Let's take a closer look at each of these possible reasons you may have gotten fatty liver…

1. Lack of movement: I promise I won't use the 'E' word, but the benefits of movement have been known for centuries. The more sedentary you are, the less you move on a consistent basis, the slower your metabolism. This raises the risk that you will develop heart disease, as well as a weight problem, which, as we know, is a prime cause of fatty liver. You know that movement also makes your circulatory system strong and reduces blood pressure, but did you know that it actually improves your liver health too?

Aerobic movement (walking, swimming, cycling, etc.) adds healthy **oxygen** to your blood. Your heart rate speeds up, and repeatedly moving large muscles invigorates the flow of healthy blood throughout your body, as well as to your liver. Aerobic physical activity also reduces your chance of becoming overweight. Strength building, especially resistance training like lifting weights or working with elastic bands will improve bone density and strength while building muscles.

Liver disease frequently attacks the bones, so when you make them stronger with strength training, you help them resist the effects of liver disease, while also reducing your risk of developing liver issues in the first place.

2. Environmental toxins: When you see clouds of exhaust leaving the tailpipe of a vehicle ahead of you in rush hour traffic, you probably roll up the windows, because who would want to breathe that? However, the toxins and poisons in your environment are not always as easy to spot. For instance, did you know that furniture and carpets release toxic gases, especially when they are new or are exposed to the light? Even many sunscreens contain compounds called phthalates. These are known cancer-causing agents which can do severe damage to your kidneys and liver.

- Phthalates are literally everywhere and have a dramatic and negative health impact on so many mental and physical bodily processes. They are found in cosmetics and fragrances, and are sometimes used to improve the flexibility of vinyl and plastic. You can find them in hairspray, skin moisturizers, soap, personal care products, the toys your children play with, food packaging and plastic wrap. They are frequently used as an important ingredient in lubricants, plumbing products, vinyl flooring, insecticides, detergents and medical devices.

- Green tea is an extremely healthy super-food you should be drinking regularly. However, *green tea extract* can actually damage your liver. The same is true for the supplements Kava Kava and Comfrey.

- Hair dye quickly enters your bloodstream through your hair follicles and can cause abdominal pain that is a signal your liver has been damaged by the chemicals your vanity has you painting your hair with. There is a reason the warnings are often twice as long as the instructions!

- You have probably heard that DEET, a toxic chemical found in some bug repellents, should be avoided. It can cause harm to your overall health and well-being, and especially your liver. Opt instead for natural and organic answers to keep stinging and biting insects and bugs away.

- Oxybenzone and Retinyl Palmitate are two other chemicals you may spot on the ingredient labels of common household products that are absorbed into your bloodstream when applied to your skin. Exposure to these and other environmental toxins raise your risk of developing fat in your liver to the point that it becomes a health problem.

- Piercings and tattoos, as well as permanent makeup, can lead to liver-damage from inks, and blood-based diseases like Hepatitis B and C.

3. Medications: Sometimes your doctor can unwittingly cause a health problem by prescribing certain medicines. Liver damage sometimes occurs as a side-effect when you take drugs and medications intended to lower your cholesterol or fight inflammation. Synthetic estrogens, paracetamol, amiodarone, and some drugs used to treat diabetes could actually be the cause of your fatty liver diagnosis.

Remember that you are a unique individual, mentally and physiologically. Some people have absolutely no problems taking a particular medication that causes a severe and negative effect on liver health in someone else. If you take long-term medications, monitor your symptoms carefully based on when you start and stop, and ask your doctor or health care provider if there are any issues with liver damage, and if so, ask if there any alternatives.

4. Recreational drugs: If you drink alcohol, you dramatically increase your risk of winding up with a fatty, compromised liver. Drinking large amounts of beer, wine and alcohol regularly can accelerate the growth of fatty liver to the point of cirrhosis, which if left untreated, can lead to death. If you take controlled substances like amphetamines and narcotics, you are also damaging your liver, and the same is true when you smoke or chew tobacco. Thanks to strong public health initiatives, you probably already know that drugs, alcohol, and tobacco are doing you harm. So, if you are still consuming any of these, it's time to get real with yourself, recognize that it's severely hurting your health, and do what is necessary to stop once and for good.

5. Family history: If someone in your family tree has (or had) diabetes or any form of Fatty Liver Disease, your risk is raised. Genetics are often a contributing factor to a number of diseases and illnesses, and this is the case with fatty liver too, especially if you have the same dietary habits as your relatives. But please don't let this feel like a curse that was placed upon you since your birth. Your family's medical history only means that you have had a higher predisposition to this problem. Reversing your fatty liver is within your power, no matter what genes you start out with.

6. Being diabetic: For people with diabetes, fatty liver creates one of those vicious circles where the symptoms of one feed the other. Diabetes is basically when the body becomes unable to manage insulin, which clears the sugar out of the bloodstream after it is eaten. Since the liver is responsible for insulin (and other hormones), having a liver that's filled with fat degenerates its ability to regulate blood sugar and metabolism.

We will cover all of these and more in the proceeding chapters. But first, let's talk about when you realized something was wrong.

CHAPTER 7

Discovering Your Trigger

The trigger on a pistol or rifle causes the gun to fire. Before it's pulled, nothing happens. But the instant that trigger has enough force exerted upon it, an explosion occurs that creates the powerful boom of a bullet going through the gun's barrel.

Your introduction to fatty liver disease may have happened the same way.

There is often a single event or factor (a trigger) which acts as the coming-out party for NFLD or NASH. You may have experienced minor symptoms in the past, but they didn't happen regularly or powerfully enough to get your attention.

Then something occurred that triggered the health situation and made you stand up and take notice. You went to your doctor, blood tests were taken, you maybe had an ultrasound, MRI, or CT scan, and eventually, you were diagnosed with a fatty liver.

Sugar: For some, the trigger is consuming a lot of sugar and simple carbs in a short period of time, leading to glucose spikes and eventually, insulin resistance. That's probably why so many people discover their condition around the holidays when their bodies are taking a nutritional beating.

Alcohol: Some people may have been drinking alcohol for years, possibly even decades, without any severe symptoms or signs there's a problem. Then one night of particularly heavy overindulgence takes their liver past the point of no return, and they start to physically feel it.

Toxins: Quite a few people experience liver problems after they do home projects like refinishing furniture, painting, sanding the deck, etc. All these (and many more) expose your liver to solvents, chemicals, dust, and fumes. If your liver is already compromised, this may be the straw that breaks the camel's back.

Trauma: A traumatic incident where your liver gets bruised, like a car accident, or a steep fall, can also lead to a weakened liver, which makes you symptomatic.

Binging: If you don't eat many fresh vegetables and fruits, and commonly enjoy processed and fast foods, after an especially monumental "pig out" session, the liver can become scarred or damaged.

Water: Stop drinking water, and your liver will eventually say, *"No more!"* A lack of hydration over even a short period of time can lead to the development of damage.

Sleep apnea: This condition results in less oxygen entering your body while you sleep. Medical News Today reported in August of 2016 that obstructive sleep apnea which contributes to low nighttime oxygen levels has been linked to a higher risk of NAFD.

Combine any of these together and add in some extra stress, and what was once just a little extra fat in your liver becomes serious enough so that it's effecting your life.

What Is Your Trigger?

It is important to identify what caused your unique situation and led to the development of your fatty liver problem. If you can trace your earliest symptoms back to an overindulgence of food, alcohol or tobacco, you are armed with powerful information.

Knowing your trigger, you can then create a lifestyle where it's easy to avoid the unhealthy habits that weakened your liver to the point of initial damage in the first place.

If you notice symptoms spike after weekend getaways or when you eat out, your body is telling you it needs help. It is practically waving a red flag and saying

"Don't do that unless you want me to become overworked and damaged, so I can't do my job properly."

Continuing those behaviors that trigger an unhealthy liver, and in due course, you could experience cirrhosis or diabetes or even cancer. When this happens, the eventual resolution sometimes means death.

Identifying your fatty liver trigger puts you in control over the situation. If you burn your hand on a hot stove, you naturally and quickly learn the lesson.

You stop putting your hand on stoves. ;-)

Identify your trigger, and you can set up the appropriate environment, eating habits and support network that can return your liver to proper health.

PART II: PREPARING FOR A HEALTHY LIVER

CHAPTER 8

Making the Commitment

Before we get into the nuts and bolts of what I did to heal myself, and how it can help you reverse your own condition, I need to ask you 2 questions…

1. Are You Ready To Feel Better?

The reason I bring it up is because unless (and until) you are ready to make significant changes in your life, your life will not significantly change. You will continue to feel worse, and your liver will continue to deteriorate.

2. Are You Ready To Let Go Of Your Past?

Regretting things you did in your past, whether it's not eating right, not moving your body, or not following a specific career path (or whatever), is a huge waste of energy.

In fact, focusing on the past keeps you from being the best you can today, and it prevents you from living in the present. Regret also promotes stress and anxiety, which can cause further inflammation in your body and your liver, and make your situation worse.

"There are better things ahead than any we leave behind." - C.S. Lewis

That's a great way to look at your fatty liver diagnosis. What's behind you has passed. You have no power to change it. You did what you did, and now you are where you are.

What good does it do to think about what could have been? Regret leads to indecision, and indecision leads to inaction. Action is exactly what you need to be taking right now, rather than dwelling on yesterday.

This very second, you are in control of the present moment. Now is the time to plot your course for the future. Look at what is ahead for you, imagine amazing health, vitality and wellness, and then **commit** to making that happen.

Better Health Begins Today

The good thing about this program is that it is highly *flexible*.

I understand that you and I are not the same, and yet, we are probably quite similar in a lot of ways. That is why I developed a fatty liver program you can adapt to your life and health goals.

Everyone is different, and you may have environmental, social, physical, or personal issues that mean your path to health and wellness are going to be different than mine.

As I mentioned in the introduction, I was diagnosed with a fatty liver in 2014, and I struggled with it for several years. Through my own journey and tons of research (and using myself as a test subject), I found out what does and does not work for me. The more I shared that with friends and people I met, the more I realized it works for others too.

I will show you exactly how I went from being diagnosed with fatty liver to a place of healing and health. This not only works, I'll go out on a limb and say it's your *best shot* at reversing your condition, if you are willing take action and do something about it.

You'll see the greatest benefits when you stop having silent *"what if"* and *"I wish"* conversations in your mind.

Look, the future is not guaranteed to anyone, but smart people plan what actions they are going to take tomorrow, next week and next year. All you really have control over is yourself, and that starts with what you do now.

Your liver is one of the only organs that can regenerate and repair itself. It wants to be healthy, it wants to be vibrant and alive, it wants to act as the filter to keep your blood clean and your digestive tract operating properly.

When you stop doing the things that kill liver cells and promote the development of health, **your liver will automatically begin to repair itself.** Make small strides at first, do what you can. Any action in the right direction deserves a pat on the back and a little happy dance.

When you notice yourself having a win, no matter how small, that one step will begin to build on the next, and you'll start confidently taking more and more of the steps and actions that will ultimately heal your body.

Free Yourself From Judgment

Move forward without judgment, from yourself or others. If you stumble along the way, no problem, just get back on the path. While your eventual goal may be an all-organic, plant based diet, it may take a while to get there, so be patient with yourself, whatever outcome you are shooting for.

Heck, you may never even go all the way, but take the first few steps, and I guarantee you'll feel (and look, and sleep, and think) better than you have in years.

There's a huge gap between eating nothing but junk food 3 times a day, and enjoying a whole-food plant-based diet that makes you feel healthier and more vital than you have been your entire life.

Find *your* place in between those two vastly different lifestyles. Anytime you can, start nudging yourself towards the former. This is *not* a zero-sum game. If you don't think you can do something completely, try to meet it halfway.

Use Pain As A Motivator

You bought this program because either you or someone you love has been diagnosed with fatty liver. Even if your symptoms are mild and occur irregularly, the pain, emotional stress, frustration, uncertainty, and fear you have can be crippling.

Use your physical and mental pain and suffering as a motivator. When you have moments of weakness, when you want a Big Mac or a Coke or a piece of cake, remind yourself how bad you feel with a compromised liver, and how you don't want to ever feel that way again.

You can do this. I don't know you personally, but I know human beings are much stronger and more capable than they can possibly imagine. I repaired my fatty liver disease and am now living a lifestyle that is full of health and happiness. I lost weight, changed my life, heck, I even wrote this program (how's that for an accomplishment).

The fact is though, I am no one special, just an average person with an **above average desire** to become healthy. That is why I say I know you can do this.

Okay, are you ready to move forward without judgment, without questioning your past behaviors, or wishing you would've done something differently? Great, look at today as the beginning of the rest (and best) of your life.

Let's get started.

CHAPTER 9

Your Liver *Hates* These Things!

If all you ever do is avoid the food, household goods, chemicals, and toxic environments listed here, you will make a **significant** impact on your liver.

The first thing I learned on my journey is that you need to stop the poisoning before you can start the healing.

There are a number of significant benefits beyond a healthy liver when you remove these toxic items from your life.

- Your brain becomes sharper
- Your senses improve (taste, smell, touch, sight, and hearing)
- You find yourself feeling less stress, anxiety, and depression
- You breathe easier
- Your joint pain lessens
- Your skin and hair begin looking strong and healthy
- You lose weight
- You start having more good days than bad

It's circular actually: The healthier and happier you are, the better your liver does. And the better your liver works, the healthier and happier you are.

A Word About Stress

I mentioned earlier how mental stress can trigger the release of hormones (specifically norepinephrine, adrenaline, and cortisol), which are hard on the liver. Of course, when that stress is short-lived, or if it's infrequent, those hormones are dissipated quickly, and your anxiety disappears. The problem is when you frequently experience severe stress.

See, your nervous system has two basic states, *sympathetic* and *parasympathetic*. The sympathetic state you are probably quite familiar with. It's also known as the "fight or flight" state, where you are always on alert, ready for trouble, never able to relax.

Nowadays that's the **default** for most people, especially those with a fatty liver. And that's a problem because it's hard on your body and even harder on your organs.

That's why you want to nudge ourselves back into the parasympathetic state, the state you are most naturally meant to be in. That is the state in which you can relax, clear your mind, and see life without the drama filter most of us unknowingly wear.

The parasympathetic state can be accessed by deeply relaxing, doing breathing exercises, movement, being in nature, and a few other things we'll talk about in a bit.

It's an easier state to enter when you are properly nourished, fully hydrated, and well rested, but regardless of where you currently are, a few minutes of deep conscious breathing will almost always clear your head and help you see things more clearly.

When you are stuck in the sympathetic state, the constant perception of a threat to your body can quickly lead to nervousness and inflammation. Your liver is already weak from an unhealthy buildup of fat. There could be scarring, and the continued inflammation from stress hormones only makes your situation worse.

Here are a few simple ideas to help change your state:

- Take up a mindfulness meditation program. Many are free and one of my favorites is listed in the index section.

- Learn how Pilates or yoga can reduce stress and anxiety in your life, and look for classes in your area.

- Whenever you notice a stressful situation occurring at work, home (or online), remove yourself from that environment as quickly you can.

- Stay the heck off Facebook, news sites, and avoid charged topics like politics with friends and family. You won't change anyone's mind, you'll just stress yourself out and harm your existing relationships.

- Don't buy into other people's drama, or let them decide your mood or outlook. Take control of your emotions, and remember, you can't control what happens in the world, but you can control your reaction to it.

You can eat all of the right foods, avoid the wrong ones, move regularly, and stay hydrated, but if you allow constant mental and emotional stress to impact your life, you can **still** do damage to your liver, and other organs too.

Foods And Drinks Your Liver Hates

Alcohol – Of all the things you ingest, the one that should be avoided *entirely*, if you have this serious condition, is alcohol. If your liver is compromised, or fatty, or if you have hepatitis, cirrhosis, diabetes, or scarring of any kind, alcohol is literally poison. Even if your fatty liver is of the non-alcoholic variety, drinking can be dangerous because it directly reduces the functionality of the part of your liver that's still healthy (the part keeping you alive). I'm not saying you can never drink again, but most of the doctors and liver experts I spoke with said you should take a break from alcohol while you are in recovery. That's what I did.

Sugar – Sugar is the main reason fat builds in your liver. It's almost as bad as alcohol. Refined foods (especially those with high fructose corn syrup) like candy, soda, desserts and baked goods are high in sugar. But even salty foods like soup, crackers, salad dressings, and chips contain sugar as we learned earlier. Juices, energy drinks, supposedly healthy cereals and condiments (like ketchup) can contain extremely high levels of high fructose corn syrup, which is not only damaging to your liver but to your overall health and well-being (plus it makes you fat). Remember to read your food labels diligently.

Fast Foods – In the movie *Supersize Me*, Morgan Spurlock actually gives himself fatty liver and pre-diabetes by eating at a well known fast food restaurant 3 times a day for a month. If you haven't seen it, you definitely should. It's a real eye-opener. My point is that the ingredients in virtually all fast foods are liver poison. Seriously. Yes, it's cheap and easy to go to the drive-thru after a long day. I get that. But this is your health we're talking about, and if you're serious about getting your life back on track, your fast food days need to end.

Processed grains – Whole grains are good, but once they are refined (processed, ground up, infused with chemicals), they wreak havoc on your body. Processed grain products include white pasta, white bread, and white rice, all of which have had a lot of the nutrition removed to make them last longer. White flour foods should also be avoided, which means cookies, crackers, snack foods, cakes and breakfast cereals. White flour is sometimes sneakily listed as wheat flour to make it sound healthier. But unless it's specifically called "whole wheat" flour, it's refined to the point where it acts **exactly** like sugar does in your body, spiking your insulin, and creating a diabetic response.

Trans fats – Food manufacturers sometimes hide these fats under other names. If you see the term "partially hydrogenated," you are looking at trans fats, which are found in many baked goods, and almost all fast foods. These force your liver to work extra hard to eliminate them, and can lead to weight gain and other serious health conditions. Trans fats are so dangerous that adding them to food is actually **illegal** all over Europe and in some US states!

Soft drinks – A number of studies show that people who regularly drink soda pop raise their risk of getting NAFLD. Just one can of soda a day can raise your odds by 45%! Most soft drinks are literally loaded with sugar, but diet soft drinks can be just as bad on your liver. Because they are sweet, diet sodas **trick** your body into thinking there's sugar in it, which means it produces the hormone insulin to clear out sugar that's not really there. That confuses your body, and can lead to insulin resistance, blood-sugar spikes, and eventually diabetes. Plus there's a link between the aspartame and inflammation. These compounds are a factor in aging and the development of many degenerative diseases like atherosclerosis, chronic kidney disease, and Alzheimer's.

Saturated fats – You should avoid saturated fats like margarine, lard, shortening, butter, mayonnaise, cream-based salad dressings, pork, beef, lamb, fried foods, cheese, and cream. If it gets hard as it cools (and especially when refrigerated), it's one of the fats to avoid. The link to diabetes and fatty liver is very real, and recent studies show that saturated fats disrupt your hormones and insulin levels, and are now an established cause of diabetes.

Foods with a high glycemic index – The glycemic index rates how quickly foods break down and turn into sugar in your body. Certain foods like potatoes, corn products, chocolate bars, white rice, baked goods (and many more) are high in simple carbohydrates, and they break down quickly, which spike your insulin and are quite hard on your liver. We will cover this in depth later on in the program.

Ice cream – The liver is not fond of dairy or sugar, and those should be avoided. But in this case, the cold temperature is also a problem. Cold foods and drinks reduce the upper intestine's temperature, and consequently, it's ability to digest food. This makes the liver work extra hard since the food isn't completely broken down when it gets there. It's like a triple whammy to your liver: Sugar, fat, and low temperature.

Some cooking oils – Soybean oil, canola oil, safflower oil, corn oil, sunflower oil all contain high levels of omega-6 polyunsaturated fatty acids, which can be harmful to your liver. Try cooking with olive oil or avocado oil instead.

Cholesterol – Cholesterol is a type of fat that is only in animal-based products. It is found in high levels in egg yolks, organ meats, shrimp and shellfish, chicken liver, fast foods, animal fats and oils, and red meats. Processed and salted meats such as bacon, salami, pepperoni, ham, pork sausage, corned beef, turkey bacon and deli meats are also extremely high in cholesterol. There is no "good" cholesterol in any food, and if you have a liver condition, you should minimize your consumption.

Too much salt – Most Westerners, and those in other countries who eat SAD diets, over-salt their food, putting high levels of sodium into their bodies. This leads to higher than normal rates of heart disease, brain disorders, dehydration, and high blood pressure, which can make your fatty liver worse.

Non-Food Items Your Liver Hates

Getting healthy goes way beyond food, here are a few liver killers you may not have considered…

Acetaminophen – If you take any type of medication for headaches or pain relief that contains acetaminophen, you could unknowingly be causing liver damage. There are 100,000 calls to poison control centers, 56,000 emergency room visits, 26,000 hospitalizations, and more than 450 deaths a year from liver failure due to acetaminophen poisoning. If you have fatty liver, ask your doctor if it's safe for you, and for alternatives of it's not.

Pesticides on/in food – Some of the food you eat may have dangerously high levels of pesticides and glyphosate (Roundup), which is poison for your liver and whole body. Avoid GMO foods, and choose organic when possible. Depending on where you live, try to shop at farmers markets and farm stands. There's nothing like meeting the farmer who grew your food.

Nonstick cookware – Nonstick pots and pans are easy to clean, but they contain polytetrafluoroethylene (PTFE) and other toxins that can contribute to liver failure, cancer, and reproductive damage. Try one of the new "green" non-stick varieties, they aren't quite as slippery, but they are a lot safer.

Plastic bottles – Bisphenol A (BPA) is an industrial chemical found in plastic products, as well as reusable and single-use containers for beverages. If you buy bottled water, you could be exposing yourself to BPAs and other toxins which are hard your liver. Brand new research even shows that exposure to BPAs can lead to fatty liver symptoms later in life, even if you live like a saint. Recent studies show that even BPA-free bottles have found to be quite toxic! Best to opt for stainless steel or glass when possible.

Some herbal remedies - Herbs like Kava Kava can lead to liver damage, hepatitis and even liver failure. It is banned or restricted in some countries but still available in the US, and often used to treat menopause symptoms. Here are a few other herbs and herbal remedies that can cause damage to your liver:

- Green tea extract
- Barberry
- Black cohosh
- Chinese ginseng
- Comfrey
- Germander
- Gordoloba yerba tea
- Greater celandine
- False pennyroyal
- Jamaican bush tea
- Jin Bu Huan
- Misteltoe
- Squawmint oil
- Sassafras
- Senna
- Skullcap

Tobacco and nicotine – Smoking does a double whammy on your liver: It acidifies your body, encouraging disease, increasing your risk of contracting lung (and liver) cancer, *and* decreases your body's ability to purge toxins. Vaping is not much better, so take a break while your liver is healing, and if you can, consider quitting all altogether.

Illicit drugs – Heroin, cocaine and other illegal drugs are damaging to your mind and body. The same is true for amphetamines, ecstasy and hallucinogenic mushrooms. Cocaine and peyote have specifically been linked to liver damage. Even though smoking marijuana may be legal where you live, its frequent use can be hard on the liver, so please abstain while you are healing your body.

Some prescription medications – Benzodiazepines, Codeine, Tetracycline, Corticosteroids, Diazepam and Temazepam are generally considered safe if you do **not** have advanced liver disease. But if you do, check with your doctor for advice and/or liver-safe options.

Chemotherapy – If you are undergoing chemo for cancer treatment, the risk of damaging your liver rises because of the negative side-effects of some common chemo drugs. Make sure you are following the correct protocol, and getting the proper nutrition (high in antioxidants) so your liver stays as strong as possible through the chemo and recovery process.

Diabetes – The presence of diabetes increases your chances of developing a fatty liver. Diabetes, due to insulin resistance, triggers weight gain in the belly, and causes your liver to store more fat. The good news is that as you start to reverse your fatty liver, your diabetes symptoms may lessen a bit.

Excessive vitamin A – The danger is not vitamin A from fresh, organic fruits and vegetables, it's from supplements. Only supplement with vitamin A if you are actually deficient, follow the recommended doses on the labels, and check with your healthcare professional for suggested doses.

Excessive iron – Your body has no way of eliminating excess iron except through actual bleeding. Like vitamin A, check with your doctor and only supplement with iron if you are actually deficient. Make sure to follow the recommended doses on the labels.

Excessive Omega-6 - Too much of Omega-6 essential fatty acid can also harm your liver. Only use supplements if you are deficient.

Polluted environment – Smog, air pollution (indoor and outdoor), and chemical exposure have a lasting effect on your liver, and not a good one. I had a friend who ended up in the emergency room because his roommate set off a bug bomb without telling anyone. He was OK, but you **know** it did a number on his liver.

Some infections or illnesses – Viral hepatitis A, B and C, autoimmune hepatitis, tuberculosis and intestinal infections caused by a candida yeast overabundance can attack your liver cells and reduce their functionality, sometimes leading to liver failure. If you have an infection and the doctor gives you antibiotics or other medications, make sure to tell them about your compromised liver.

Miscellaneous Liver-Killers Found Around The Home

Ammonia, air fresheners, fabric softeners, antibacterial products, bleach and other household cleaners, kitchen and window cleaners, chemical herbicides, fertilizers and insecticides, sprays for killing ants, roaches and other bugs, paint, paint thinner, carpet cleaning products, and any chemical found in and around your home can pose a risk to your overall health, and can irritate your fatty liver.

Whenever you use any harsh chemical household product, cleaner or solvent, wear gloves, long sleeves, and eye protection. If you are working inside, consider using a respirator that covers your mouth and nose.

Healthy Alternatives To The Chemicals Your Liver Hates

You have options when it comes to chemicals and toxins, and as someone who cares about their liver, you should regularly seek them out:

For Sun Protection

- The best plan is to simply wear more clothing. Pants, glasses, hats, and long-sleeved shirts go a long way to protecting your skin.

- If you can, avoid direct sunlight from 10 AM to 2 PM, which is when it's at it's strongest and most dangerous.

- For those times when you must be outside, use a sunscreen with natural mineral barriers and no chemicals or hormone disruptors. My favorite line is *Blue Lizard*, also available on Amazon. Another good one is *Vanicream*. Both of these brands cost more than other sunscreens. But if you have liver issues, you don't want to use cheap crap on your body because it's absorbed through your skin, gets into your bloodstream, and eventually, winds up in your liver.

- Some oils have a surprisingly high *natural* sun protection. Red raspberry seed oil has an SPF of 28 and protects against UVA (and UVB) rays. Carrot seed oil has an SPF of 38, wheat germ oil is 20, and even high-quality coconut oil has a natural SPF of about 5. Best of all, none of those will harm your liver or overall health.

- Antioxidants, specifically from food, can help heal and repair damage and are ultimately going to be good for the skin. You won't block the sun, but you will recover faster. Foods with carotenoids, green drinks, vitamin C or E are also great for your joints, heart, eyes, and brain, and help with fatty liver symptoms.

For Mosquito and Bug Repellent

- Make sure that standing water is removed from around your house (buckets, pots, gutters) since that's where bugs like mosquitos breed.

- Mix 32 ounces of apple cider vinegar with 2 tablespoons each of dried rosemary, lavender, thyme, sage, and mint. Shake before using in a spray bottle and apply to your skin.

- Mix water with peppermint oil (about 30 to 1) and citronella oil (about 40 to 1) and spray around the outside of your house (doorways, windows, eaves) to repel bugs like ants, roaches, and silverfish.

- Use citronella candles and oils outside to repel bugs and mosquitos without sprays or poisons.

- Consider an electric bug zapper, which kills bugs with electricity instead of chemicals.

Makeup, Skin and Hair Alternatives

- Many cosmetics are made with preservatives or chemicals, which can leach into your body and damage your liver. Look for natural and organic lines that are non-toxic. Sites like *Sephora* have entire lines devoted to Natural Cosmetics.

- Coconut oil is an excellent body lotion and dandruff fighter. It keeps your skin healthy and strong, prevents it from drying out, and reduces the chance you'll develop wrinkles.

- The fleshy leaves of the aloe vera plant make an excellent skin moisturizer and softener, and their antioxidant qualities can heal skin damaged by the sun. (I like to mix some in with my morning smoothie as well because studies have shown it to be so good for you.)

Natural Alternatives to Chemical Cleaning Supplies

- Add a couple of teaspoons of tea tree oil to filtered water for a natural disinfectant that destroys fungus on all your household surfaces.

- Mix 1 teaspoon of cornstarch, several drops of your favorite essential oil, and 1/4 cup of white vinegar with 1 quart of warm water. This makes an excellent glass and window cleaner, especially when you use crumpled newspaper to wipe dry. Paper towels may cause streaking.

- Baking soda is a natural deodorizer. It's excellent for scrubbing and light cleaning. Add 1/4 cup of baking soda to a 16 to 24-ounce spray bottle for an excellent general cleaner.

- Add 1/4 cup of lemon juice and one cup of hydrogen peroxide to 12 cups of water. This makes a natural all-purpose cleaner. Add a couple of drops of lavender oil for a wonderful smell and calming aromatherapy benefits.

CHAPTER 10

Your Liver *Loves* These Things

There is an old saying…

"You catch more flies with honey than you do with vinegar."

I assure you this is true. You'll get more of what you want when you are sweet than when you are sour, and positive reinforcement usually works better than negative reinforcement. Think about it. Would you rather be told what you *can't* do, or what you *can* do?

Most people prefer to be rewarded, rather than slapped on their hand and told *"No!"*

We just talked about a bunch of the things your liver does not like. Looking through that list you might have encountered some of your favorite foods, or a household product you regularly use.

Knowing those items can damage your body, even make your fatty liver worse, might have depressed you a bit. Hey, I get it, it was no fun giving up foods I loved my whole life, but I figured out how to re-engineer my diet, and in some cases, replace things I *had* liked with things I now love.

Helping Your Body Become Alkaline

The following foods, beverages and lifestyle practices all make your liver smile. Many have a high nutritional value, and they also support optimal pH levels.

pH refers to the amount of potential hydrogen in your body. It's one indicator of how healthy you are. The higher your body's pH reading, the more alkaline and oxygen-rich your blood is. When your pH reading is low, it means your body has become acidic.

When your body becomes too acidic, it's more difficult for you to absorb minerals and other nutrients. You often feel low-energy, your cells do not naturally repair themselves, and your ability to eliminate heavy metals, toxins, and poisons is reduced. You may become more susceptible to illness, infection and disease.

The pH scale starts at 0 and moves all the way up to 14. The normal human range for human blood is very narrow, around 7.35 to 7.45. The **optimal** alkaline level of a robust and healthy liver is 7.4, or just slightly alkaline.

You can test your own pH, to monitor your progress, with specifically formulated (and inexpensive) test strips available at Amazon.

The human body normally does an **excellent** job of regulating it's own pH, which means you probably don't need to think about it very much. However, when you eat acidic foods, specifically sugar and alcohol, you put yourself at a disadvantage.

When you enjoy an optimal pH measurement in your liver and body, all of your organs work together with the rest of your processes for the best possible health. and alkaline.

Foods Your Liver Loves

Consider this the "short" list of foods that support and heal your liver. In the diet section (Chapter 15), we will review these and many more. We'll also talk about how to integrate them into your daily meal plans.

Cruciferous vegetables – Of all the foods you can eat, probably the most powerful, available, and affordable are cruciferous vegetables like broccoli and cauliflower. The active ingredient is sulforaphane, which is beneficial for liver health, losing weight and even fights cancer. Broccoli, cabbage, arugula, brussel sprouts, collard greens, and bok choy are all cruciferous vegetables that contain sulforaphane.

Leafy greens – Spinach, lettuce, and kale are probably the leafy greens you are most familiar with. They contain fiber, and help your liver neutralize chemicals, pesticides and heavy metals that may have arrived in your body attached to the foods you eat. Chard, arugula, celery, mustard greens and turnip greens also qualify. There are many ways to eat these greens besides salads. You can have them steamed, sautéed, in stirfrys, and in soups and stews.

Carrots and beets – The flavonoids in beets and carrots specifically boost the overall effectiveness and functions of your liver.

Turmeric – The incredible healing properties of the curcumin contained in turmeric can help with joint, organ, and muscle pain. This is one spice you can add to many savory recipes, including stirfrys, vegetable juices, soup, even tea.

Whole grains – Processed grains like white flour are bad for you because of the way they break down in your body, but **whole grains** are quite good for you. My favorites are oatmeal, quinoa, brown rice, farro, barley, and buckwheat. You can eat them for breakfast, lunch, or dinner, as a main or a side dish.

Legumes - Kidney beans, black beans, mung beans, navy beans, chickpeas, lentils and split peas fill you up, give you energy, are full of healthy fiber, and promote liver health. They are satisfying, high in vegetable protein, low in fat, and contain nutrients and minerals your body needs. Most Americans are severely deprived of legumes, even though they are one of the most powerful foods in existence!

Apples – That old saying *"An apple a day keeps the doctor away"* might just be referring to liver doctors. Apples are super high in pectin, a chemical that promotes your liver's detoxing and filtering process.

Berries – Berries are like little food gems rich in antioxidants, vitamins, and minerals. If you have a sweet-tooth, they are a nice treat because they can satisfy you without spiking your blood sugar or harming your liver.

Green tea – Excellent for your liver health because of antioxidants and compounds known as catechins. Work this into your daily routine, and sip on Green tea while you think positive thoughts.

Walnuts, pumpkin seeds, and other nuts – Walnuts and chia or pumpkin seeds contain high levels of omega-3 fatty acids, fiber, as well as glutathione, which boosts liver health.

Artichokes – Artichokes are part of the thistle family, and are an ancient natural liver and blood cleanser.

Tomatoes – Raw tomatoes do an outstanding job of detoxing your liver. When cooked they still provide liver-boosting properties, but raw, organic tomatoes are preferred. There's a great gazpacho recipe in the diet section of this program.

Asparagus – Loaded with healthy dietary fiber that helps pass waste through your system, it also promotes liver health, and it tastes great too.

Garlic – Garlic has selenium and allicin that cleanse the liver, and other components that flush out toxins.

Citrus (Lemons, Limes, Oranges, and Grapefruit) – Not only are these foods high in vitamin C and antioxidants, but they also make your liver's job easier and can reduce inflammation.

Avocado – The avocado is a superfood. Eating ¼ of an avocado every day delivers over a dozen minerals, nutrients and vitamins your body craves.

Sprouts – Sprouts are an excellent source of protein and chlorophyll, which helps the liver's filtration process.

Herbs that heal – There are specific herbs with liver-healing benefits like milk thistle, dandelion and burdock root.

Digestive enzymes – We will cover enzymes in detail in the supplement section. Personally, I take papaya extract before every meal, and on cheat days (or whenever I eat animal protein), I also take a proteolytic enzyme that helps break it down.

More Things Your Liver Loves

Movement - You should be getting 90 minutes a day of movement, which most people can find the time for when they give up their social media addiction. ;-)

Aerobic movement strengthens your heart muscles. This means that you pump blood throughout your body without much effort. Your pulse slows down because it's not blocked, and your blood flow improves. That makes the delivery of blood to your liver much easier than if you did not enjoy aerobic physical activities.

Strength training is the most efficient physical activity for building muscle. You burn fat, calories and carbohydrates for up to 48 hours after a strength training session. You probably recall from our earlier discussion that being overweight and obese is a leading cause of fatty liver. Strength training is an excellent fat burner and your liver loves it.

Gentle, non-pounding aerobic activities like walking, cycling and swimming are less intensive forms of physical movement you should focus on while you are healing your fatty liver. Gentle is the key, because as you remove toxins and poisons from your body, you could feel a little weak or *"out of sorts."*

A properly hydrated body - Your body can go without food for around a month as long as you are getting water into your system. But if you are not hydrated, after about 5 days, you will be knocking on death's door. Your body needs water for many important physiological processes to take place. This includes keeping your liver happy.

Think about it this way, the largest and heaviest internal organ is your liver. The human body is 60% to 70% water. It doesn't take a math genius to realize that water would be extremely important to the hardest working organ in your body.

A properly hydrated body helps your liver remove waste, assists your liver in removing toxins and poisons from your body, and promotes healthy blood flow to and from your liver.

Laughter – I thought I'd throw this one in there because the physical and mental healing properties of laughter are utterly amazing. When you laugh, you produce an antibody that helps in the first stage of defense against bacterial infection. This means laughing cuts down on the amount of toxins your liver has to deal with, and when you laugh you generally feel good about the world. Positive emotions like happiness and contentedness reduce your stress levels, meaning less inflammation in all your organs.

Love Your Liver

The rule of thumb is that vegetables, fruits, legumes, nuts, fruits, and whole grains lead to a more alkaline state, which helps your body heal itself. On the other hand, meat, dairy, refined grains, sugars, and alcohol, create a more acidic state, which creates more inflammation.

You want the former, rather than the later. Let your healing start now, and watch the pain dissipate until it's finally gone.

CHAPTER 11

Mindset And Avoiding the Negative

Becoming a healthier, stronger "you" might also require eliminating toxic people <u>and</u> situations from your life. This includes the physical and virtual, as well as mental and emotional places you spend your time.

Getting off Facebook, ignoring gossip, and minimizing the depressing 24 hour news cycle leads to far less stress and anxiety. Staying away from negative people, places and things, as well as situations that are filled with anger and worry, is absolutely crucial to reversing fatty liver disease and enjoying total wellness. Remember that stress hormones create inflammation, and make your body acidic.

Reducing The Negative Influences In Your Life

The average person spends an astonishing 2 hours a day on social media websites. Do you think that you could cut that time down, and instead invest your new-found time walking, meditating, cycling, or clearing junk foods from your pantry?

Maybe even visit a Farmer's Market, or cook some delicious veggie soup, or prepare some meals for the week ahead?

I guarantee that time would be more rewarding if spent on something positive, like enjoying people you know and love: Parents, close friends, children, grandchildren, or other quality individuals.

Avoiding junk-food junkies

While we are at it, let's mention another problem, which is spending time with people who have poor dietary habits. If your favorite co-worker loves fast food, or has a candy fixation, or simply can't eat a salad every now and then, that's someone you want to take a "break" from.

If you are particularly close, try to spend time with them that doesn't involve eating. I have a friend like that, and whenever she says we should do "happy" hour together, I suggest taking a hike, or going to the beach, or something healthy instead.

People with bad diets tend to influence us, and make it seem like it's OK to poison ourselves (and harm our liver). It's not!

When they are constantly saying things like "It's only one ice-cream cone" or "everyone has fries with their burger," it means they don't take their health seriously. And if they don't care about **their** health, they certainly aren't concerned with **yours**.

Remember, *you* are the one who will pay with soreness, a foggy brain, extra weight, and other fatty liver symptoms. You are the one who will suffer the increased risk of liver scarring, cirrhosis, and cancer, not them.

Finding your inner strength

As human beings we make excuses for our actions. The next time you find yourself having to create a reason to justify some negative behavior… just… stop…

And remember yourself when you were truly suffering.

It makes no sense to tell yourself lies if the end result is a lower quality of life. Remember, your main reason for getting healthy and keeping your liver (and other organs) highly functional is so you can live without pain or other symptoms.

Dig down deep into your mind - and emotions - for the true reason you are about to do something that will harm your recovery, and stop it dead in its tracks.

Choose some action or activity that either promotes health and nutrition, gets you physically active, boosts your brain and emotions in a positive way, and otherwise produces a positive result that will not cause further damage to your liver.

The only thing you truly control is
what you think and what you do

Try to catch yourself when you are making food decisions, and take the time to consider the potential outcome. When you do that, you have a good chance of making a positive choice instead.

It feels good to take control of your life and develop the confidence that promotes making more smart choices in the future.

CHAPTER 12

Movement

Getting your body active and moving doesn't have to take place in an intimidating and sweaty gym. You can stay physically active throughout the day, just about anywhere, whether at work or play.

When you are healing your liver, the key is to focus on minimally intense activities, but do them for longer periods. A simple 60 minute walk, preferably in nature, can help calm your mind and gets your body moving. Walking is a perfect healthy liver activity. It's low stress and low impact, but it increases your heart rate enough so that your body benefits.

Studies show that walking **regularly** can have as much of a positive effect or in some cases, even more benefit than running! The same is true for yoga, tai chi, swimming and resistance routines that are also low impact.

What Are Some Simple Ways You Can Keep Fit?

Body weight training uses the weight of your own of body and resistance to strengthen your muscles and promote mobility, heart health, positive mental function, and many other benefits.

Sit-ups and push-ups are examples of body weight movements. If you have ever squatted down to pick up something off of the ground, bending your knees and lowering your upper body, you have promoted proper health with a form of body weight training.

As you can imagine, you can do this kind of work out at home, or anywhere you like. Just pick a small number of repetitions to start with, and little by little see how much further you can go.

Create opportunities for movement throughout your day

- Instead of hiring a neighbor kid to mow your lawn, do it yourself. Not only will you get your blood flowing, you'll save some money too.

- Get out in the garden and do some weeding, which helps you stretch and get some fresh air.

- Call a neighborhood friend and tell them you can walk over for a cup of tea, rather than having a conversation on the phone while you lounge on your sofa and eat some junk food.

- Better yet, make it a habit that every time you are on the phone to get up and walk around. You won't even notice that you're on the move because you'll be nice and distracted by talking and listening.

- Walk to a Mall or shopping area near you, or if it's far, park a few blocks away. In fact, you can add this little trick, and always park away from the entrance a bit. You'll squeeze in a little movement, and often find it's much easier to find parking too!

- If it's just a few floors up, make a habit of always taking the stairs instead of the elevator or escalator.

Those are just a couple of examples of opportunities for physical activity all around you. The following list will give you some more ideas about how to add movement to your daily routine.

- Join a hiking or walking club. If there is not one in your area, start one with some friends.

- Go bowling once a week.

- Walk around your neighborhood first thing in the morning, after hydrating, but before you reach for your coffee. Then the coffee feels like a reward.

- Write it down. You write your doctors appointments and child's soccer games on your calendar. Why not do the same for your movement schedule? This simple trick changed everything for me.

- Buy or rent bikes for the entire family and go on family cycling trips and picnics.

- Make a plan to hike or walk all of your city's parks and trails, and get to at least one every weekend.

- Do you live in a cold winter climate? Just 30 minutes of shoveling snow from the driveway burns 182 calories. Sledding burns 205 calories, and ice-skating 191 calories in the same time frame.

- Get out of your office chair and do a few squats when you are standing throughout the day.

- Start taking a short 10 or 15-minute walk after dinner. This aids your digestive process, improves circulation, and makes it easier for your liver to do its job properly.

- Whenever you find yourself walking anywhere, alternate your pace from brisk to casual. You can tell the difference as your breathing changes, and you'll be amazed how much energy this gives you.

- Buy a stationary bike or treadmill and use it while you are enjoying your favorite TV program, which actually makes watching television healthy!

- Clean your house or garage. Not only will you move your body, but you'll create a clean environment for yourself. Move clutter out of your life, just like you are doing with your body.

- Schedule a fun and physically active day at the beach or a park.

- I bought a light set of dumbbells at a garage sale, and keep them near the front door, where I see them before my daily walk. You'd be surprised at how much more they get used when they are constantly visible.

- Put a yoga mat next to your bed. This will promote a healthy yoga practice every morning, and right before you go to bed.

- Replace your coffee break at work with a 10-minute walk to a fresh juice bar or have a cup of herbal tea.

- Purchase a pedometer or set up your smartphone and aim for 10,000 steps a day. Even 5,000 steps a day is excellent if you are just starting out.

- Attach a resistance band to your bathroom door knob. After mother nature calls, spend a few minutes on some quick strength training.

- Instead of asking someone else to fetch something, get up and do it yourself, every time, even if someone else is closer to what you need.

How long should you engage in physical activity?

Ideally, you should be getting 90 minutes a day of physical activity. You don't need to work out hard for 90 minutes straight. You can mix it up over the day.

I take a 45-minute walk every morning, and try to go to the gym for 30 minutes in the afternoon. I also spend at least 30 - 45 minutes a day working in the garden, walking around town, visiting a neighbor, or taking an evening stroll.

If all this is new to you, relax and take your time. Try and get as close to 90 minutes a day of movement as you can, and just do your best. I recommend committing to 10-minute chunks. Most people can do just about anything for 10 minutes. ;-)

Can 10 Minutes of Movement Really Provide Noticeable Benefits?

If you don't think that short bursts of physical activity do much for your overall health and well-being, consider this: One study had a group of women split their fitness sessions into 10 minute increments. A second group of women kept moving for 20 to 40 minutes at a time.

Incredibly, the first group of women lost more weight, got healthier and stayed that way after 5 months, and were more likely, than the second group, to enjoy physical movement consistently!

Another study that will blow you away and change your ideas about how powerful physical movement is was conducted at the University of Virginia. Men and women of different fitness levels were asked to complete 15 exercise routines each week that only lasted 10 minutes each.

After 3 weeks, those volunteers showed aerobic fitness levels equal to that of people that were 10 to 15 years younger! Also, flexibility, strength and muscular endurance were equal to that of men and women 20 years younger.

The big takeaway here is that you don't have to run marathons and train to become an Olympic bodybuilder to get yourself in awesome shape.

Avoid "all-or-nothing" mindsets that rationalize if you don't have an hour, you may as well not get active at all. If you only have 10 minutes to take a jog, go for a swim, enjoy a brisk walk, or hit the bicycle, it's worth it.

CHAPTER 13

Supplementation

The truth is, people with very healthy diets and lifestyles usually don't need much, if any, supplementation. They get what their body requires *naturally* from the food they eat.

That's why this program focuses on diet as opposed to supplements.

But for some of us, our bodies are so deficient, or inflamed, or damaged, that we need something extra, especially if our livers are severely compromised.

1. There may not be enough nutrition in our food. It could be we are eating junk, or maybe our liver isn't able to process the nutrients that are present because of it's weekend state.

2. Our lifestyle is depleting our body of nutrients faster than they can be replaced (from alcohol, smoking, stress, toxins, etc.), which creates deficiencies.

3. We need extra supplementation to deal with specific issues (like pain or digestion).

I personally use several supplements, but before you run off and spend hundreds of dollars at the vitamin store, or online, or anywhere else, there are a few things I recommend you do first...

•   Ask your doctor to order a full blood panel to see if there's anything *specific* you are deficient in. Blood tests can catch quite a few nutritional problems, not to mention elevated liver enzymes, cholesterol levels, and other abnormalities.

•   Discuss the supplements you are considering with your doctor. You can even show him this book with the list. Make sure there aren't any potential problems (allergies, interactions, etc.) with existing medications you already take.

•   Begin slowly. The list below is in order of importance to give you a starting point. If you are new to supplementation, perhaps just begin with a probiotic, digestive enzyme, and some Milk Thistle, and add in what you feel comfortable with down the line.

•   I recommend you either buy your supplements direct from the manufacturer, from a trusted source like Amazon (with multiple reviews), or from a local supplement store so you can support your community. Avoid discount and grocery stores since many of the supplements they sell are low quality.

- Always get the highest quality products you can afford. It amazes me how many people will spend $200 on a pair of jeans, but they'll buy the cheapest possible supplements, which are going inside their body.

- Always follow the dosage information from your doctor or health care professional, otherwise, follow the instructions on the label of the supplement itself. Double the dosage does *not* mean double the benefits!

In the case of a damaged liver, whether you have inflammation and scarring or not, the following supplements may help speed up your recovery, and some even help prevent liver disease from the get-go.

1. Probiotics - I'm convinced the best way to start your day is to drink a cup of warm lemon water, eat something that's probiotic (or take a probiotic supplement), and go for a walk. Foods like kimchee, tempeh, and sauerkraut are great, even some miso soup, which is part of a traditional Japanese breakfast. If you are feeling ambitious try something like Beet Kvass before your walk.

For people who want to take a supplement instead, there are quite a few shelf-stable probiotics available online and at your local health food store. In several studies, probiotic supplements that included *bifidobacterium bifidum* and *lactobacillus plantarum* improved liver function in those with various diseases and conditions. That makes sense because probiotics help your digestive tract **break down** the food so it can be utilized more effectively by the liver.

2. Enzymes - Another thing that really helped out my liver is taking digestive enzymes with every meal, especially meals where I ate a lot or consumed meat. Enzymes such as amylase and lipase are supportive of the liver. Betaine hydrochloride (HCL) is believed to fight inflammation. Proteolytic enzymes and papaya enzyme supplements support healthy digestion.

Some of my favorite brands are...

- *Now Papaya Enzymes*, which is a good broad-based enzyme that breaks down just about everything.

- When I'm eating meat or a heavy protein meal, I also take *Premier HCL* supplement, which helps my body fully digest it.

- During my cleanse, I take *Dr's Best Proteolytic Enzymes* first thing in the morning, and an hour before dinner.

3. B-Max - It is believed that once the liver has been scarred, it won't regenerate itself. That's why it's so important to pay attention to your body so you can take care of any problems as they come up. However, if scarring has already occurred, B-complex vitamins can help with the effects of cirrhosis, like memory loss, nerve damage, and inflammation. I take *Premier B Max*, which helps with energy management, stress, organ detoxification, heart health, and mood balance as well.

4. Milk Thistle - Milk thistle is a well-known herb for overall liver health that has been used for thousands of years. It's generally safe, effective, and can also keep many liver problems from worsening once they are diagnosed.

As functionality starts to deteriorate, a dose of 200 mg of a milk thistle supplement taken 2 - 3 times each day may be effective for rejuvenating and repairing liver damage. Look for standardized 80% silymarin content. The brand I use is *Jarrow*.

5. Curcumin and Turmeric - You can take a daily curcumin supplement (my favorite is *PuraThrive* at Turmeric.us) or you can simply add turmeric spice to your meals, smoothies, fresh juices. Widely regarded for its preventive and healing benefits this wonder-herb has been linked to strong heart health and slowing down the aging process, as well as protecting liver cells from fat-infestation. Incidentally, no other herb has been clinically tested or written about as frequently for its inflammation-fighting properties. Since a fatty liver and other liver problems usually have inflammation as a symptom, it's a great addition to your supplement regimen.

Studies have shown when you add black pepper to turmeric, you increase the bioavailability of the curcumin by as much as 2,000%, which means it's more easily absorbed by your body. You can sprinkle a pinch of freshly ground black pepper on your turmeric right before eating to get the most out of this super-spice or purchase curcumin capsules with piperine, the active ingredient in black pepper. Later in this program, I'll give you my recipe for Golden Milk, which you can make at home (it's delicious). If you have aches and pains, it's a great way to enjoy your daily turmeric.

6. Dandelion Root - Often combined with milk thistle in supplement form, dandelion root provides iron, potassium, and zinc which support liver functionality. This natural healer also helps bile production and the easy transference of bile between the liver and gallbladder. Dandelion root chunks can be used for the DIYer to make a healing tincture or tea, or to include with a smoothie.

7. Magnesium - There are many great benefits from magnesium, but for liver sufferers, it helps to normalize blood sugar and blood pressure, keeps your immune system functioning properly, helps with the creation of protein, and it is involved in heart, nerve, muscle, and liver function. An added benefit is that it also helps with constipation and sleep issues. I like *Trace Minerals Liquid Ionic Magnesium* best since I can add it to my lemon water, smoothies, and juices. We also recommend eating almonds, tofu, and spinach which are excellent natural sources of easily absorbable magnesium.

8. Burdock Root - Burdock root can be purchased as a supplement, and also in rough-cut root form at some natural health and grocery stores. The roots can be used in juices and smoothies, and to make a tea which is a common blood purifier in Ayurvedic and Chinese medicine. Just like the dandelion root, burdock root stimulates bile flow while helping a weak liver purify and filter blood, and restore damaged cells to health.

9. Artichoke extract - Artichokes can be eaten with a low-fat plant-based dip, or you can take an artichoke extract supplement that contains cynara. That's the active ingredient in artichokes that does what so many liver-friendly supplements do, it stimulates healthy bile production and flow. It also prevents gallstones and can reduce the symptoms of jaundice. Tinctures can be made from dried artichoke leaves or flower buds.

10. Vitamin E - Vitamin E is a powerful antioxidant. Oxidant stress due to insufficient oxygen levels in the liver promotes scarring and the development of diseases like fatty liver. In some studies, vitamin E delivered significant improvements in the health of liver tissue versus the quality of liver tissue before a daily vitamin E supplementation was started. A good friend of mine with fatty liver swears by vitamin E, saying it was the only thing that helped him. We also recommend eating tomatoes, avocados and healthy nut butters which are excellent natural sources of easily absorbable Vitamin E.

11. Vitamin C - You should be eating berries, brussel sprouts, and citrus fruits as a natural source of easily absorbable Vitamin C. If you need more, or if your doctor recommends it, doses as low as 500 mg of a Vitamin C supplement help prevent fatty buildup, and reduce your risk of developing cirrhosis. Vitamin C also helps flush fat from your liver and has been shown to strengthen the immune system and help ward off disease.

12. NAC - N-acetyl cysteine is a powerful supplement that directly supports the removal of toxins from your liver. In fact, if you overdose on acetaminophen, they'll give you NAC via an IV in the emergency room, it works that well, providing protection against harmful free radicals throughout your body.

Supplements that contain NAC should not be taken for an extended period of time, as they have been known to contribute to kidney stone development after frequent and continued use. I take it only during my cleanse, and never for more than 4-weeks straight.

13. Rhodiola - Recent studies show this little-known supplement stimulates muscle energy and glycogen synthesis in the liver, as well as speeds recovery due to damage. Rhodiola regulates blood sugar levels (for diabetics) and protects the liver from environmental toxins.

For many, supplements are the extra boost that helps them finally start healing their fatty liver.

Be aware the only things I personally take on a **day to-day** basis are probiotics and digestive enzymes. The others I take for a month or two, or when I am actively cleansing.

CHAPTER 14

Putting It All Together

The liver is able to regenerate itself, even after it has been damaged. When you think about it, that's pretty amazing. It means that in some cases, abuse that happened over many years (or even decades) is reversible.

That's not the case with most organs: When your heart or kidneys or brain start to go, that's pretty much it. But the liver is truly unique in that you can stop poisoning it and start supporting it, and **it will begin to rebuild itself**.

For 80% of the people reading this program, you can reverse your fatty liver disease with a few simple dietary changes. Thousands have done it before you. It just requires the right information about diet, the right knowledge about toxins, a positive mental attitude, and a sincere desire to feel better.

You can take control of your life, I promise that. I did, and I'm certainly not the most disciplined person (ask my wife).

For me, the shift happened when I finally had enough. I simply couldn't take the pain and depression anymore. I was tired of looking and feeling like junk, and always being too exhausted to leave the house. One day, after dragging myself out of bed, I looked in the mirror and said "No More!"

Don't beat yourself up about whatever it was that got you to this point, that's in the past. Instead, resolve to start *paying attention* to what you eat, how often you move, and the environments (and people) you voluntarily expose yourself to.

That's the first step, and the hardest one… deciding to finally wake up and take responsibility for your health.

Let's Recap Where We Are

When you add all 5 pillars of the **Fix Your Fatty Liver** program to your life, you stand the best chance of reversing your condition totally.

That means none of the physical pain and mental frustration and anxiety you are going through right now have to be a part of your future when you get totally on board with the 5 pillar approach…

1. Proper Diet and Nutrition
2. Creating A Healthy Environment
3. Positive Mindset

4. Physical Movement
5. Supplementation

Your body wants to be healthy. The human body is miraculous in its ability to heal and promote human existence, even if we do negative things to it.

Ancient Chinese and Indian healers believed that the liver is the key to total health, that a healthy liver can even overcome other shortcomings in your body to help you live a full and vibrant life. I completely agree.

What you learn in this program is based on modern-day research, science, and medically approved methods but also employs Ayurvedic and Traditional Chinese Medicine practices that lead to the healthiest liver possible.

PART III: FATTY LIVER DIET

CHAPTER 15

The Fatty Liver Diet

Unless you are poisoning your liver with alcohol, or exposing yourself to dangerous chemicals, or are **genetically** predisposed to having a fatty liver based on your family history, you probably got your condition from your food.

In an overwhelming majority of cases, food is the **primary** cause of fatty liver, specifically if you eat what we refer to as the Standard American Diet (SAD). And while that sounds like bad news, it's actually good news because food can also be the **solution** to your problem.

This section of the program is the longest, and as far as I'm concerned, it's the most important. In fact, if you only read one thing, this is it. Follow the right diet, eat the healthiest food, and chances are, it will make the biggest difference to your health.

The Fatty Liver Diet outlined here is the **same** food plan I used to reverse my condition and heal my body. It's 100% natural, affordable, evidence-based, and in many cases, scientifically shown to help you overcome your disease, provided you haven't progressed to something more serious.

And even if you have, it's probably the best opportunity to get yourself healthy again **without** expensive drugs or the side effects that come with them.

Benefits Of The Fatty Liver Diet

Here are the biggest benefits people experience when they implement this…

1. Faster, easier weight-loss.
2. More natural energy, without spikes and crashes.
3. Healthy, regular bowel movements.
4. Falling to sleep quickly, sleeping soundly, waking up easily.
5. Better digestion and less gas.
6. A sharper, quicker, faster brain, and more mental clarity.
7. Fewer aches and pains in your joints and muscles.
8. Smoother skin, and in some cases, a reversal of skin conditions that have plagued you for years.
9. An overall feeling of wellness that must be experienced to be appreciated. You feel peaceful and tranquil most of the time, in control of your emotions and feelings

Your Relationship With Food

Before anything else, let's talk about complex relationship many of us have with food, which may be a problem in and of itself. For quite a few people, food is about **much more** than nutrition or fuel.

In fact, our earliest memories are often about food and eating…

- Baking cookies with our family (and licking the bowl afterward)

- Dinners on Sunday evenings

- Getting sweet treats because we were well-behaved

- Eating in the cafeteria at school

- Going out to restaurants

- Being denied food because we were bad

- Being forced to eat everything in front of us

- And many more.

A lot of those memories are connected to emotions we may find either very satisfying or very unpleasant, which is why so many of us have trouble staying at a healthy weight.

You see, because of the **emotional** connection we've had with food our whole lives, the food ends up controlling us, instead of the other way around. It's like we are hypnotized by our stomachs.

Have you ever found yourself…

- Eating because you feel **depressed** or empty inside?

- Feeling **angry** with yourself because you ate too much in one sitting?

- Feeling **guilty** because you didn't finish everything on your plate?

- Eating certain foods because they remind you of a time in your past when you were **happier**?

- Cooking or preparing something because it makes you **feel** a certain way?

- Overeating (or over-drinking) because of **social pressure** you experience from friends and family.

- Giving yourself permission to eat unhealthy food because that's how **other people** around you are eating?

- Finding **mysterious** candy or junk-food wrappers in the trash, not remembering when you ate the product that came in them?

- **Bingeing** and then **starving** yourself, perhaps over and over again. Then feeling guilty every time you do?

I have personally experienced every one of these, and the reason why is because food is extremely powerful, especially the way it **makes you feel** inside and the memories it can trigger.

Food actually has the power to activate specific emotions like guilt, happiness, anger, sadness, exhaustion, excitement, even shame. There's been quite a bit written about the term "emotional eating" the past few years, and one of the best books is by our friend Dr. Glenn Livingston called *Never Binge Again*.

(Glenn is offering a free copy for customers of **Fix Your Fatty Liver**, see index in the back.)

If you are an emotional eater, especially if you have trouble following a healthy meal-plan or staying on a diet (regardless of which diet it is), I encourage you to do some work in the area of emotional eating.

Until you do, the best diet in the world won't do you a bit of good because you probably won't stick to it. You need to take the time to figure out your own unique relationship with food and identify (and break) old patterns that may be keeping you overweight and making your liver sick.

6 Tenets Of The Fatty Liver Diet

OK, let's talk about the Fatty Liver Diet and how it's different from others you may have tried in the past…

There are **many** kinds of diets out there, hundreds in fact. Each one is designed with a very specific outcome in mind. Some are meant to help you gain weight and build muscle, some are meant to help you burn fat and get slim, and a few are meant to treat a specific condition like acne or eczema or joint-pain.

The Fatty Liver Diet was specifically created to help **support your liver**, dissolve fat, and heal your body from the inside out. The philosophy behind this diet is that your liver is the most important organ since it controls just about everything else:
- Regulates hormones

- Burns calories
- Filters toxins
- Digests food
- Controls your mood
- Regulates cholesterol
- Cleans your blood

Now listen, you will absolutely lose weight on this diet, in fact, I lost over 30 lbs, and I've kept it off for over a year now. But this is **not** a specific weight-loss diet. That means you will lose weight gradually as opposed to burning fat immediately.

Rapid-weight loss diets have their place, but **not** if you have a compromised liver.

In fact, many of the low-carb, high-fat diets like Atkins or Paleo can actually be **dangerous**, even if you are otherwise healthy. They are not something you want to do long-term.

On the other hand, the Fatty Liver Diet helps you develop **good eating habits** that not only clean up your liver but also help you regulate and control your weight and vitality forever, all while giving you the nutrition you need to stay healthy and happy.

This program allows you to sustain yourself forever, which is why I call it a "diet for life," as opposed to a quickie fix that only works for a little while.

There are 6 principles of the Fatty Liver Diet:

1. Whole Food Plant Based (WFPB)
2. Organically Produced
3. Encourages Alkalinity
4. Low Glycemic Index
5. Supports Healthy Gut Bacteria
6. Satisfies Hunger

Let's look at each of these:

1. Whole Food Plant Based (WFPB)

The first tenant is that we want to eat whole, *minimally processed* foods that are derived from plants, which means we avoid things like junk food, crackers, cookies, as well as meat, poultry, and fish.

Listen, I'm not trying to go all vegan on you. I have always **loved** steak and eggs, salmon, chicken, and other animal protein, and I occasionally indulge. But if you have a fatty liver, and you want to actually **get better**, you are going to want to take a WFPB approach to your diet and cut out animals for a while.

I did, and in about 90 days, I'd almost completely reversed my damage. I'm convinced that the animal protein (and saturated fat) was causing much bigger problems that I realized. If you are willing to stick with it for a few months, I'm betting you will see similar results.

I'm not saying you can **never** eat meat, but remember that every time you do (especially when you are trying to heal yourself), you're going backward, and potentially harming yourself all over again. At the very least, take a break and see how you feel. Add it back gradually, and pay attention to how you feel afterwards.

The Problem With Eating Animals

The evidence that meat is dangerous for fatty liver sufferers is pretty compelling…

1. Meat contains saturated fats that are hard to digest and can spike your blood sugar, creating a diabetic response in your body, which harms your liver, kidneys, and heart. It's difficult to digest, and putrefies inside your colon, creating chemical reactions that can increase likelihood of fatty liver and even cancer.

2. Most meat is factory farmed and pumped full of dangerous hormones and antibiotics, which can also damage your liver and alter your internal hormonal balance.

3. Worst of all are the heavy metals, chemicals, pesticides, and herbicides that are in the animal's food, and that are **passed up the food chain to you** when you eat them. Even organic grass-fed beef may have these chemicals in them, so don't think you are safe because you are eating "clean."

The WFPB approach is generally healthier than eating meat and processed foods. Kaiser Permanente (the health insurer) also released a great free handout (link in the index) that talks about how to transition from eating meat to eating mostly plants.

2. Your Food Should Be Organically Produced, And Always Non-GMO Certified

Genuine organic foods are usually healthier than non-organics because they are grown without pesticides or chemical fertilizers. All of those things can stay on the food, even if it's washed. They enter your body through the digestive tract, and ultimately harm your liver and contaminate your blood, which is already compromised.

While there's no real science that proves GMO foods are dangerous in and of themselves, there is **plenty** of evidence that **the way they are grown** *is* dangerous. Many GMO foods are engineered to be resistant to herbicides, specifically glyphosate, which is used in the growing process.

The problem is that glyphosate gets into the food on a cellular level and then actually enters your bloodstream. It's toxic for all humans, but it's **especially** damaging for people who have fatty liver.

In fact, it's been specifically linked to NAFLD and fatty liver symptoms. Which wouldn't be a problem, except that a whopping 93% of all urine tests performed by the University of California came back positive for glyphosate.

So while we highly encourage you to stick to organic food when possible, we absolutely **do not recommend** eating anything that may be genetically modified, especially GMO corn, wheat, or soy, or anything grown with herbicides like glyphosate.

3. Foods Should Encourage Alkalinity

When your body becomes too acidic, you begin to lose the ability to absorb minerals and other nutrients. You lose energy, your cells do not repair themselves, and the ability of your liver and the rest of your body to detoxify heavy metals, toxins, and poisons begins to weaken dramatically.

One of the best ways to keep your body alkaline is to eat foods that are fresh, nutritious, and in their natural, unaltered state. You want to avoid **anything** containing alcohol or sugar, or processed foods like cookies, cakes, or crackers.

4. Foods Should Have A Low Glycemic Index

Speaking of processed… The glycemic index refers to how quickly a particular food breaks down in your body and **turns into** sugar. In this case, lower is better.

For example, a bowl of steel cut oats has a glycemic index of 42 but a bowl of puffed rice cereal has a glycemic index of 82. Both the oats and the rice puffs have about the same number of calories, but the oats break down **much slower** in your body and give you energy for **many** hours. You won't become hungry or get low blood sugar from the oats. In fact, they are a nearly perfect food for fatty liver sufferers because they are fulfilling.

The puffs taste good going down, but the rice flour they are made with **immediately** turns to sugar (plus it has added sugar), and that spikes your insulin. That means you'll have a **serious** sugar crash in about an hour, and will become hungry, needing to eat, and starting the domino effect all over again.

Typically the more ground up and processed your food is, the faster it breaks down in your stomach, and the higher it's glycemic index. On the Fatty Liver Diet, you want to eat things that will help you stabilize and normalize your blood sugar. There's a great site to check the glycemic index of your foods in the back of this book.

5. Supports Healthy Gut Bacteria

The bacteria in your gut is known as your biome. This biome helps break down food in the upper intestine so your liver can separate the good from the bad, and eliminate the waste.

Probiotic supplements have their place, but there are probiotic (and prebiotic) foods that encourage a healthy gut biome in a natural and low impact way. These can aid your digestion, and make bowel movements easier, and more regular.

I eat things like sauerkraut, kimchee, pickled cucumber, and lots of greens in my diet to keep my biome healthy and keep things moving. ;-)

6. Satisfies Your Hunger

The most important thing of all is that a diet must **satisfy your hunger** or you will not be able to stick to it, and you'll go back to your old way of eating.

You should **never** feel hungry on the Fatty Liver Diet, or any diet for that matter. If you are hungry, it means you aren't eating enough of the good stuff, or you are consuming things like sugar, processed food, or alcohol, which are throwing your body out of whack and messing up your blood sugar.

Portion Control

One of the big problems with most diets is they have complicated rules about how much you can eat, breaking things down into weights and measurements, or giving points to certain kinds of food.

When something is complicated, people don't do it. That's why I want to differentiate this diet from others you may have tried, and say if you are eating based on the above guidelines, you **don't need strict portion control** or a food scale.

Eat healthy, and you can eat till you are full, and enjoy yourself without worrying if you ate an extra ounce of oatmeal or drank a large smoothie when you meant to make a medium one.

It's more about filling yourself up with healthy stuff, and sticking to ratios than it is about watching your overall quantities. For example, you shouldn't just eat endless amounts of rice, because that means you're not getting your fruit and vegetables. But if you're getting enough of each, go wild. None of the foods on our *good-to-eat* list will hurt you, they are all healthy and infinitely better that what you were probably eating before (especially if you were eating processed foods).

And for the record, I think you should occasionally cheat with a small portion of something you used to eat, if only to see how the "old" food makes you feel. But if you are like many people, you won't want to go back to your old food, because it will probably taste way too sweet or salty.

The great thing about the Fatty Liver Diet is that every step leads to the next. When you eat a whole-foods-plant-based-diet, especially if it's organic, you are already consuming low-glycemic, high-alkaline, healthy-gut foods.

Eating this way has a huge number of benefits, and it creates a Positive Cycle which actually makes the change easier. And best of all, because we focus on food **quality** as opposed to **quantity**, we are no longer worried about how many ounces or bites of food we are eating.

What Are The Specific Foods Of The Fatty Liver Diet?

In this section, we'll review the most healing, healthy, and important foods for people who have a fatty liver. Many of these are **scientifically** shown to have a positive impact on liver health, and all are an important part of my own diet.

1. Cruciferous vegetables

Of all the foods you can eat for a fatty liver, probably the most powerful, bioavailable, and affordable is broccoli. I literally eat it 1 - 2 times a day, raw, steamed, and sautéed, in large part because it's so good for my liver.

One well-known study showed that eating broccoli powers up the functionality of your internal enzyme system to help your liver get foreign molecules, toxins, and poisons out of your body. And another one revealed that **sulforaphane** (the active compound in broccoli) is beneficial for losing weight and may even fight cancer.

Broccoli, cabbage, cauliflower, arugula, kale, brussel sprouts, collard greens, mustard greens, radish, turnip, and bok choy are all cruciferous vegetables that contain sulforaphane. They are extremely versatile and can be used in many healthy dishes and recipes.

2. Whole grains

My favorites are oatmeal, quinoa, brown rice, black rice, barley, bulgur, farro, rye, and spelt. Whole grains fill you up without harming your liver. In fact, there's pretty solid evidence that oatmeal specifically helps with fatty liver, and can reduce inflammation.

You can eat whole grains for breakfast, lunch, or dinner, and they make a great side dish or base for a stirfry, even a healthy addition to a salad. Organic non-GMO whole wheat is OK in moderation, but if you must have bread, stick with those made from sprouted grains.

I try to avoid corn because much of it is contaminated with pesticides and herbicides that can damage your liver, but if you know for a fact it's genuinely organic, you can treat yourself occasionally.

3. Legumes

My 3rd favorite fatty liver food is beans and legumes… Kidney beans, black beans, mung beans, navy beans, chickpeas, lentils, and split peas fill you up, give you energy, contain a lot of fiber, and promote liver health.

They are also highly satisfying, full of vegetable protein, low in fat, and contain nutrients and minerals your body needs. Not to mention they are a low glycemic-index food and tend to break down slowly, helping you regulate blood-sugar, and achieve optimal body weight, all things your liver appreciates.

Last but not least, beans stop the recycling of toxic bile that your liver has already processed, which can improve digestion and further encourage weight loss.

4. Leafy greens

Leafy greens have some cross-over with cruciferous veggies (like collard greens and arugula). Both help your liver neutralize chemicals, pesticides and contaminants that may have arrived in your body attached to the foods you eat.

Spinach and lettuce are probably the two leafy greens you are most familiar with, along with kale, chard, arugula, celery, mustard greens and turnip greens. Herbs like cilantro and parsley are great blood tonics that help your body eliminate heavy metals as well.

5. Turmeric

The incredible healing properties of the curcumin contained in turmeric were discussed in an earlier section. This is definitely a food item your liver loves because it stimulates the production of bile and helps your body digest and process fats properly.

It is also considered an anti-inflammatory agent and a detoxifier. Great for joint-pain, a sore liver, and general aches and pains.

I like to cook with fresh turmeric 2 - 3 times a week, juice with it, add it to smoothies and make what's known as "Golden Milk" that helps reduce joint pain. I'll give you a recipe for that later in this program.

6. Apples

That old saying *"An apple a day keeps the doctor away"* might just be referring to liver doctors. Apples are super high in pectin, a chemical that promotes your liver's detoxing and filtering process.

My two favorites are the Fuji and the Granny Smith. Both are delicious, make a great snack, and help fill you up between meals so you don't feel like eating junk. I love having dessert after dinner, but I know that many sweets are not good for me, so now I have an apple, which is satisfying, and a LOT healthier than a brownie or ice-cream.

7. Berries

Berries are rich in antioxidants, vitamins, and minerals. If you have a sweet-tooth, they are a nice treat because they can satisfy you without spiking your blood sugar or harming your liver.

Treat yourself to strawberries, blackberries, blueberries, raspberries, and if they are available, try some of the more exotic varieties like acai berries, acerola cherries, cranberries, goji berries, salmonberries, boysenberries, or ollalieberries.

8. Other Fruit

Stone fruits (plums, peaches, nectarines, fruits with a pit), melons, and bananas are full of vitamins and minerals. Many have a slightly higher sugar content (and glycemic index) than apples or berries, but still have a lot of fiber, which means they are ultimately healthy.

If you have a sweet tooth, try to satisfy yourself with fruit before reaching for a candy car. Fruit contains fructose, but unlike High Fructose Corn Syrup (HFCS), it doesn't spike your blood sugar because of all the fiber.

9. Green tea

Freshly made green tea is excellent for your liver health because it contains antioxidants and compounds known as catechins. Steer clear of green tea extract in pill form though, and stick with the real stuff you brew yourself. Green tea extract can actually harm your liver.

9. Probiotic and pre-biotic foods

Eating things like kimchee, sauerkraut, and pickled vegetables help your digestive system function better, and consequently, support your liver. They encourage the good bacteria in your gut to grow, which helps your body digest and absorb the nutrients in your food, turning them into something you can actually use.

10. Walnuts, pumpkin seeds, and other nuts

Walnuts have been specifically linked to better heart health, increased bone density, and lower instances of metabolic syndrome. They can even help with diabetes.

But other nuts and seeds (pumpkin seeds, chia seeds, almonds, brazil nuts) are also healthy since they have omega 3s and other essential fatty acids. Chia and pumpkin seeds contain fiber, as well as glutathione, which boosts liver health.

11. Ground Flax Seeds

Flax delivers healthy dietary fiber that helps your system eliminate waste. It also prevents your hormones from creating a problem in your blood supply, even those unhealthy hormones which have been added to some food.

When you get flax or flaxseeds in your diet, you ensure the liver can filter your blood properly, and produce enough bile to help you move dangerous toxins out of your body. I like to add a tablespoon of ground flax in my morning smoothie.

12. Artichokes

Artichokes are part of the thistle family and are an **ancient natural** liver and blood cleanser. I like to eat one a week. They are fun, and if you have fatty liver, can be beneficial. Mix some curry powder with a little vegan mayo for a healthy and delicious dip.

13. Tomatoes

Tomatoes do an outstanding job of detoxing your liver. When cooked they still provide liver-boosting properties, but raw, organic tomatoes are preferred. There's a great recipe for gazpacho later in this program, it's one of my favorite healthy soups, easy to make, and delicious. But most of the time, I just eat them raw with a little olive oil and balsamic over them.

14. Cucumbers

Loaded with healthy fiber and antioxidants, cucumbers are cooling to your system. They can help relieve inflammation, rheumatic conditions caused by excessive uric acid, and support liver health. I use them in juice, smoothies, and also cut up with a little rice vinegar and sesame seed oil for flavor. Tastes great too.

15. Sweet potatoes

Sweet potatoes are rich in Vitamin A and also contain fiber and Vitamin C, as well as other cleansing and immunity-boosting nutrients. They have a higher sugar content than white potatoes, but are a lot healthier.

16. Coffee

I have gone back and forth as far as recommending coffee because it can acidify your body, which may lead to increased symptoms and susceptibility to disease. However, at this point, the evidence seems pretty compelling that a couple of cups of black coffee every day (without cream or sugar) is, in fact, good for your liver.

If you are a coffee lover, and you were worried that you might have to give it up, it's fine in moderation provided you don't add sweetener and dairy. If you usually use cream and sugar, try a little coconut milk and stevia instead.

17. Asparagus

Loaded with healthy dietary fiber that helps pass waste through your system, there's also some new science that shows asparagus not only supports good liver health, it may even relieve the effects of a hangover.

Of course, you shouldn't be drinking any alcohol, but the fact that it can help liver function is reason enough to add this to your diet.

18. Carrots and beets

The flavonoids in beets and carrots are excellent for your liver and blood, and beets have specifically been shown to increase your stamina and athletic performance, improving the endurance of triathletes.

I like to make a juice with both of them together, along with some garlic and turmeric. It's delicious, and it's great for you too (the recipe for that is in the juicing section of this program).

19. Garlic

Garlic will not only keep Dracula and the cast of Twilight away, but it is also great for you. It has selenium and allicin that cleanse the liver, and other components that activate liver enzymes and flush out toxins.

Cooking makes it milder but can degrade its therapeutic benefits. I like to juice it and also pickle it raw in vinegar (and keep it in my fridge). That makes it easier to eat and keeps the beneficial enzymes intact.

20. Citrus Fruits

Not only are citrus fruits high in vitamin C and healthy antioxidants, but they also make your liver's job easier. In the case of grapefruits, oranges, tangerines, and other sweet citrus, make sure you're eating the actual fruit and not just the juice. That way you get the fiber, which helps reduce the blood sugar spike from the fructose.

Lemons and limes are also full of antioxidants and can be juiced to add to smoothies, teas, and warm water. I drink a warm water lemon-juice drink before I start my day, and I believe it makes a big difference.

21. Avocado

The avocado is a superfood. Eating ¼ to ½ of an avocado every day delivers up to 25% of the top 7 minerals, nutrients and vitamins your body craves. Not to mention that avocados are very filling, and many people find them delicious.

One of the many wonderful components of the avocado is an antioxidant called glutathione, which specifically helps your liver filter out harmful materials and waste products.

22. Sprouts

Sprouts are excellent. I like broccoli, sunflower, mung, barley, alfalfa, and other micro-greens. They provide excellent protein and chlorophyll, which helps the liver's filtration process. Juice them (especially wheatgrass) and you can almost feel the life-force entering your body.

23. Herbs that heal

There are specific herbs with liver-healing benefits. Milk thistle is the king of the liver-lovers and has literally been used for thousands of years. Dandelion and burdock root are two other herbs you can add when juicing or cooking, or take as a supplement to promote a strong and healthy liver.

24. Digestive enzyme helpers

I take papaya extract before every meal, and on days when I don't follow the diet 100%, (like whenever I eat animal protein), I also take a proteolytic enzyme that helps break the food down. But you can also just eat enzyme-laden foods papaya, ginger, and miso soup as a between meal snack.

In today's world, we eat so many prepared meals, that some of these fruits, veggies, legumes, and grains might not be things you normally consume. Give yourself permission to try something new, and discover food you otherwise wouldn't experience.

Cooking (and gardening) aren't a big part of our daily lives anymore, so many of the ingredients are foreign to us.

Challenge yourself to find a vegetable or bean that looks interesting, and read up on it, maybe start with a small portion. I did that with Garbanzo beans, and now they are a regular part of my diet!

The Daily Dozen

Incorporating these foods into your daily diet is actually pretty easy. I really like to follow the Daily Dozen philosophy of the NutritionFacts.org Web site. That way, I know I'm getting everything I need to stay healthy.

As we talked about earlier, portion control is not really necessary if you are eating veggies, fruits, legumes and whole grains. The key is to get the right ratio.

Every meal, you want half your plate to be veggies and fruits, one quarter to be legumes, and one quarter to be whole grains.

The Daily Dozen philosophy is a bit more specific, and I highly recommend checking it out. But if you slip up, or otherwise mess up on the ratio, don't worry, tomorrow is another chance to get back on track.

Great Meal Ideas

There are a number of different meal types I like to create, and I have listed them below based on time of day I usually eat them. Think of these like a menu that you are choosing from every day when you open the fridge and try to figure out what to eat.

Breakfast:	**Lunch:**	**Dinner:**
- Oats	- Salads	- Salads
- Fruit Bowls	- Wraps	- Stir Frys
- Smoothies	- Soups, Stews, and Chili	- Roasted Veggies
- Veggie Juices	- Veggie Bowl	- Veggie Burgers

There are so many ways to expand this list, especially because most of these foods are tasty any time of day. When you add some good snacks in, and mix up the variety of ingredients, you'll find it will take you quite a long time to exhaust this list!

Breakfast

1. **Oats** - Organic oatmeal or steel cut oats are an excellent way to start your day. Avoid the instant stuff, and instead, cook it yourself. Throw some fruit on there, with nuts, flax, nut milk, cinnamon, and a small spoonful of honey or maple syrup for a complete, healthy, and filling breakfast that will carry you through all the way to lunch without having a sugar crash.

2. **Fruit Bowls** - I love oatmeal, but I also just love to make a plain fruit bowl with apples, bananas, papaya, grapes, and some walnuts or flax. I don't do dairy anymore (and I don't recommend it), but if you must use yogurt, stick with an organic unsweetened type and just use a small amount.

3. **Smoothies and green drinks** - Probably the easiest morning food you can make is a smoothie because you just throw a bunch of fruit and nut milk into a blender, and voilà do have a happy healthy meal that fortifies your body, supports your liver, and

is easy to digest. There are some great smoothie recipes later on in this program, including my favorites.

4. **Veggie Juices** - When I talk about veggie juices, I'm talking about freshly made juices that are mostly green vegetables (60% or more), and that you either buy from a juice bar, or make yourself. Because most of the fiber is removed in the juicing process, these should be consumed primarily during your cleanse, or when you also eat them with whole fruits and vegetables.

Lunch

5. **Salads** - I like to get a few heads of kale and lettuce on my weekly shopping trip, and then every few days, chop them up and put them in the refrigerator so they're ready for a salad. This can be eaten whenever you like, but my favorite time is lunch. I'll throw some nuts, veggies, even a piece of fruit like a chopped apple or peach in there, and it makes for a complete and delicious meal.

6. **Wraps** - Another substantial lunch idea is to have a wrap. Pick up some sprouted tortillas from the health food store, and fill them with hummus, raw and roasted veggies (peppers, spinach, zucchini, cucumber, etc.), and enjoy. You can also make a sweet version of a wrap with almond butter and banana. If you want to use bread, try to stick with sprouted grains, which are less processed, and healthier than normal bread.

7. **Soups, Stews, and Chili** - At least once a week, usually on the weekend, I like to make a big batch of veggie chili, a stew, or vegetable soup. That way I have something available to eat throughout the week, or whenever I want a healthy snack. You can add beans, rice, and nearly unlimited vegetables to soups and stews to create fulfilling, balanced meals that will support your liver and help you maintain a healthy weight.

Dinner

8. **Dinner Salads** - I make my dinner salads a little heavier (and more savory) than I do for lunch, including roasted veggies, tofu, nuts, or grains. I love barley, farro, or quinoa, which adds even more fiber and makes the salad quite filling.

9. **Stirfrys** - One of my favorite go-to meals, especially for dinner, is to throw a mess of veggies into a pan with a little bit of salt and olive oil and make a big stirfry. You can put this in a bowl over rice, quinoa, or other whole-grain and make a complete meal

filled with fiber, nutrients, and protein. Add some beans and hot sauce to give it a Mexican flavor.

10. **Roasted Veggies** - An alternative to a stirfry is to roast the veggies in the oven for 20 - 30 minutes, which gives them a richer flavor, especially broccoli and brussels sprouts, Roasted cauliflower actually tastes meaty, and is very satisfying. Serve over rice or quinoa.

11. **Veggie burgers** - Another great meal idea is to make a veggie burger, which you can cook in a pan, or even on the grill. I add tomatoes, lettuce, and a pickle for flavor. When I'm feeling the need for cheese, I'll even stick a slice of nut-cheese on there for extra flavor.

Snacks

12. **Flatbread** - You can take a sprouted tortilla, and use it as the base for flatbread with pesto, veggies, nut-cheese, and other tasty items. Or you can make your own crust from whole grain flour so you know there's no junk in there.

13. **Veggie sticks** - One of my favorite easy snacks is to cut up some carrot and celery sticks, and put them in a bowl in the fridge. That way whenever I open the refrigerator door to see what's inside, it's easy enough to just grab a handful of veggies and some hummus dip or almond butter.

14. **A piece of fruit or veg** - One of my favorite fruits is an apple, which is full of liver-loving pectin, filling, sweet, and satisfying. I like to rotate my fruits based on what's in season, which can mean grapes, stone fruit, kiwi, or anything else that's interesting in the produce aisle or the farmers market.

One amazing thing I noticed is that when I shifted my diet to more healthy food, and stopped drinking alcohol, eating processed grains, and especially eliminated sugar, my body literally stopped craving those things.

Of course, it took about a month for me to really break the worst of my bad food habits, and a few more to lose my taste for those foods, but once I did, I couldn't imagine going back to the old way of eating. There's no way I would want to experience the symptoms and problems I was having before.

The Truth About Protein

Since I don't recommend eating meat or dairy on the Fatty Liver Diet, you may be wondering about protein. That's a question I get from friends, do I get enough protein from the non-meat items I consume?

One of the things I learned on my quest to get healthy was that **unless** you are a bodybuilder or an athlete, or you train physically for over an hour a day, you probably need a lot less protein than you think.

In fact, the protein in **plants** is actually superior to animals because it's easier for our bodies to process.

Most people get **far more** protein than they need, and many of us actually get too much, especially since we aren't getting enough fiber to balance it out.

Consider this, the average man needs only 3 - 4 ounces of protein **per day**, and women need even less. Now, remember that foods like beans, rice, even broccoli are loaded with protein, and you'll understand why the average vegetarian gets far more protein than required, even though none of that is from animals.

How To Cheat Without Killing Yourself

You may be wondering how strict you need to be as far as this whole diet thing in concerned. The answer is you only need to be **strict** if you want to get **better**.

I am being serious, if your fatty liver isn't a big problem, if your liver enzymes aren't elevated, if you aren't in any real pain, I suppose you could eat what you want without any immediate consequences. But I'm guessing that's not the case, otherwise, why would you be reading this?

So the answer is that you should be as strict as you can be, and try to **really stay** on the program and get yourself healthy. However, in the real world, temptation rears its head, which is why I came up with "diet cheats" that give you a bit of flexibility.

A "diet cheat" is the ability to **occasionally** break your diet, and have a little something that you normally wouldn't. Remember, your cravings will start to dissipate over time as you eat less junk, but you may find yourself thinking about some old food you haven't had in a while.

For example, I love baked goods, and one of my friends makes the most incredible brownies you've ever tasted. Unfortunately, brownies do not work as far as the Fatty Liver Diet is concerned. They contain sugar, flour, eggs, butter, pretty much everything you want to avoid.

And so, for the first few months when I started, I mostly stayed away from her because I didn't want to be tempted. Nowadays though, when I have her over, and she pulls out a few of her brownies, I will indulge.

But, I don't have a **whole brownie** covered with chocolate sauce and ice cream like I used to. These days I'll take one her brownies and cut it into quarters. Just one small piece gets me satisfied.

Same thing with desserts. Instead of eating an entire Snickers bar like before, I switched to **much healthier** dark chocolate, and just need a small piece to satisfy me.

Heck, I'll even treat myself to a cheeseburger every now and then (without the fries) and then I usually find myself just eating half of it!

My cheat strategy…

- Don't give yourself a whole cheat day, give yourself a small cheat "event" a few times a week. That means you eat 3 healthy meals, and then occasionally treat yourself to a piece of brownie or a cookie after dinner.

- See how much you can fill yourself up on vegetables and fruits, beans and whole grains before you get to the cheat item.

- Control your portion sizes on cheat items. Maybe split the burger with your spouse instead of eating the whole thing. And sub the fries for a salad. Just eat a small piece of the chocolate or a half a cookie.

- If you are going to do a big cheat (like eating a cheeseburger) get yourself fully hydrated so you aren't famished when you sit down to eat. And remember that just one seriously unhealthy meal can throw your body out of whack for a few days, so get ready to feel funky for a bit.

- Pay close attention to how you feel afterward. Eating sugar gives me a crash, and eating too much meat definitely slows me down for a day or two. Realizing that your physical feelings and emotions are affected by what you eat is the easiest way to stay on a clean diet.

There are only two strict things I never cheat with, soda pop and alcohol. Both of those are so bad for you and so dangerous to your liver, they are on my avoid-at-all-cost list.

CHAPTER 16
Controlling Your Environment

When you are in a stressful or toxic environment, you don't feel good. You suffer mentally and physically. Being constantly exposed to stress-filled surroundings can cause chronic, long-lasting problems.

The opposite is also true.

When your environment is filled with the people, places, and things you love and enjoy, the air you breathe, the liquids you drink, and the foods you eat are all positively influential, you feel and look great, and enjoy good health.

Merriam-Webster defines *environment* as:

> 1 – The aggregate of surrounding things, conditions, or influences; your surroundings.

> 2 – Regarding ecology, the air, water, minerals, organisms, and all other external factors surrounding and affecting a given organism at any time.

> 3 – The social and cultural forces that shape the life of a person or population.

Look around yourself right now. What do you see? What do you hear and smell? What is your body coming into contact with?

Everything you see, smell, touch, hear and taste, as well as anything in your immediate surroundings can affect what you are thinking and how you are behaving. This can include any number of things that factor into your mental and physical health and well-being, and influence your actions.

Start With The Shopping List

Since poor nutrition is the leading cause of fatty liver, your **shopping list** is the perfect place to start getting control of your environment. I mean, if you don't buy it, you can't eat it, right?

Look at the foods and beverages in your pantry, refrigerator, and freezer. What do you see? Are there are a lot of processed items, frozen foods, sweet snacks? Things with refined sugars, dairy, high levels of salt, and other unhealthy ingredients known to antagonize the liver?

If so, take control and replace all of those unhealthy, processed, chemical-laden products with healthy foods and drinks. Opt for things that are fresh, organic, and plant-based like fruits, vegetables, nuts, beans, and whole grains.

Have a purge, and dump the old, unhealthy junk from your life. Yes, that's right, I'm saying:

Throw it all away!

Don't worry about "wasting" food if it's something toxic or it contributes to your fatty liver. Things like that should be **thrown away** as soon as possible, they really have no place in your home or life. If you feel bad, give them to your local food bank, but get them out of your home and don't buy them again.

As you learned from previous chapters, you are actually causing your body physical harm when you eat things that are bad for you. But when you make the room for good, take control of your pantry and especially your grocery list, you ensure you'll always have **healthy food** around when you're hungry.

Your shopping list also extends to non-food items you now know can harm your liver. Hair dye, bug repellent, sunscreen and other household products should be replaced with healthy options. There are always alternatives, whether you are shopping for food or consumer goods.

Learn to read ingredient labels, know what you're putting in, on and around your body, and only buy food, cosmetics, cleaners and other goods that are **not** going to cause fat build-up in your liver.

Being Your Own Cook

Where you eat is almost as important as what you put into your body. If you frequently eat in your car, at a fast food restaurant, or casual dining establishment, you are not in control of the food you consume. How is it prepared? Where is it from? Chances are your server, or the drive-through employee you order from, has no idea what goes into the food they are serving you.

But when you cook for yourself, you control the environment, process, and ingredients. There's no way you are going to use unhealthy items, or add a bunch of unnecessary sugar, if you make something yourself.

Of course, the biggest complaint people have is that shopping and cooking take time. While that's true, you might want to track how many hours a day you spend on online, and allocate some of that for shopping and food prep instead.

Taking Your Time

Most people eat way too fast. This encourages overeating because you fill up before you feel full and then end up eating too much. That's why I recommend taking your time, and allocating at least 20 - 30 minutes to eat a meal, especially lunch and dinner.

Eating quickly can also lead to other issues, like Irritable Bowel Syndrome, digestive problems, and general inflammation. Much better to take small bites, and spend the time to **fully enjoy your food** as opposed to wolfing it down without thinking about it.

I like to schedule my meals at a specific time of day. That way I know I'll have plenty of time to eat, and make sure I don't eat too late. I recommend you eat your evening meal before it gets dark, and at the very latest, before 7:00 PM. Eating late at night can leave you feeling bloated and fat, and actually prevent you from getting a good night's sleep.

Who Are You Eating With?

Human beings are social creatures, and while we all like to think of ourselves as independent beings, we are **heavily influenced** by others.

You can't always control the "who" of your environment because you may have to eat with family or co-workers. But whenever you can, eat with people who practice good dietary practices, people who put health and happiness first, and encourage you on your food journey.

These are often people who make you smile when you see them entering your immediate area. You should also be consciously limiting your exposure to people who make you think negative thoughts, practice poor health habits, promote stress and anxiety, and bring you down.

This also needs to be addressed if you are a loner, and prefer to spend most of your time by yourself. There is nothing wrong with enjoying your own company. However, countless studies show that loners and hermits tend to live shorter, unhealthier lives than those who socialize more frequently.

Spending time with the **right** people can relieve stress and anxiety in your body and your mind, which leads to a healthy liver.

What Media Do You Consume?

Media makes up a large part of the human environment these days. Screens (monitors, tablets, computers, smartphones, smart watches, televisions, etc.) are everywhere.

Whatever type of content you consume, delivered by your favorite device, has a definite influence on your attitude, your behavior, and your outlook. And that can ultimately effect your health.

Spending time on Facebook or watching intelligence-robbing "reality" TV shows does not serve you. In fact, studies show that **Facebook and other social media sites can be a major source of stress, anxiety, even depression**.

Your favorite TV shows, songs, and movies are definitely a part of your environment, and they can positively (or negatively) impact your mental well-being. Choose carefully, since negative, violent, depressing, stressful, or sad things can alter your state and throw you off your diet.

Try to watch fewer "screens" overall, and when you do, fill those screens with positive, uplifting messages. Look for good news, happy stories, inspirational posts.

Engineering The "Perfect" Environment

Unfortunately, perfection doesn't exist in human endeavors. This means that if you wait for the planets to align, you might be waiting forever.

You should be consciously affecting as many aspects of your environment as possible. At the same time, you should learn to accept what you can't change, and **change everything that you do have control over** (which is more than you'd think).

CHAPTER 17

Smoothies And Juices

Which is better, smoothies or juicing? It's a good question. While I love a **fresh pressed** veggie juice, and it certainly has a **lot** of nutrients, I prefer smoothies for my day-to-day meals because…

Juicing removes 95% of the fiber, which means you consume more calories while feeling less full. That encourages over-nourishing, which is hard on the digestive system.

Fiber is important because it contains phytonutrients and mass, which help regulate blood sugar levels. It also aids in digestion and the creation of bile, which is how the nutrients get from the food into your body.

Sweet fruit juices (like orange and apple and carrot), contain a lot of sugar, which can actually harm your liver, the opposite of what you are trying to achieve.

The biggest issue is that people don't juice correctly. They use the wrong ingredients, drink the wrong amounts, juice too frequently, and end up consuming way too much sugar.

In this chapter, I will reveal how I use juicing, and also cover something I like even better… Smoothies!

Smoothies are a **lot** easier than fresh-pressed juice. They cost less money, and the clean-up is faster, so you are more inclined to make them. Plus, they have all the natural fiber and mass of the whole fruit or vegetable, which is a lot better for you.

What Is A Smoothie?

A *smoothie* is a thick beverage you make in a strong blender (like a *Vitamix* or *Ninja*) that contains raw fruits, vegetables, and a bit of liquid (like water) so it purees properly. You can also add things like ice cubes, protein powder, tofu, flax seeds, or even avocado for flavor and texture.

Some smoothie recipes call for regular milk or yogurt, but I recommend **replacing** those with almond (or other nut) milk since you want to avoid eating dairy when you have a fatty liver. If you do decide to use dairy, keep the amounts to a minimum, just a spoonful of yogurt at most.

Why Are Smoothies Healthy?

Of all the things you can eat when you have liver issues, smoothies are actually one of the best because…

1. They are very easy for your body to digest as they contain all the natural fiber and the blending action breaks down the ingredients to make it easy for your liver to process and absorb the nutrients.

2. You can include many of your daily dozen foods into a single meal by adding them to your smoothie. Things like nut milk, berries, and greens go down easily and fortify you until your next meal.

3. Instead of the big mess you get with juicing (or cooking), you just throw everything into the blender and in a minute or two, you have a tasty treat.

4. Recipes are easily doubled so you can make these for the whole family for breakfast or a mid-day snack.

Favorite Smoothie Recipes

The beauty of smoothies is they are extremely versatile. You can make them with almost any fruit or vegetable, fresh or frozen. If you have a powerful blender, just toss everything in, turn it on, and in about a minute, you have a beautiful meal that is healthy and delicious.

Below are some of my favorite smoothie recipes. Feel free to alter these to your own liking, you can add protein powder, sweeteners like honey or stevia, spices like cinnamon, and even supplements like B Max or Magnesium.

Each recipe makes approximately two 12 oz smoothies. Feel free to adjust or increase amounts based on serving sizes or if you prefer one ingredient over another. If you don't finish, just put in the fridge for later.

1. Morning Glory - This is my favorite go-to morning drink, chock full of vitamins, minerals, and protein. I usually make it for breakfast, lunch, or a mid-meal snack.

- 1/2 banana
- 1/2 papaya, seeded and peeled
- 1 cup of fresh or frozen berries (strawberries, blueberries, or blackberries)
- 1/2 cup greens (kale, spinach, collard greens)*
- 1/2 cup water
- 1 tablespoon ground flaxseed
- 1/2 thumb sized portion of ginger root

Blend on high for 60 - 90 seconds. *You can replace the greens with a quality green-drink extract like Organifi. Serves 2.

2. Beautiful Berry Blast - Power packed with lots of vitamin C, rich in antioxidants for inflammation relief and healthy skin. This one gives you a natural burst of energy and is great in the morning as well. Serves 2.

1 cup strawberries
1 cup blueberries, pitted cherries, or raspberries
1/2 green apple
1/2 cup greens (kale, spinach, collard greens)
1/2 cup water
1 tablespoon fresh lemon juice
1 tablespoon ground flaxseed
1 thumb sized portion of turmeric

Blend on high for 60 - 90 seconds. *You can replace the greens with a quality green-drink extract like Organifi. Serves 2.

3. Protein Power Punch - Great for before or after you do your daily movement, this also makes a nice dessert treat or afternoon snack. Feel free to add some unsweetened chocolate powder for extra flavor.

1 banana
1 cup unsweetened almond or soy milk
1/2 tablespoon honey or maple syrup
1/2 cup greens (kale, spinach, collard greens)
2 tablespoons vegetable protein powder (like Vega)
1 tablespoon ground flaxseed
2 ice cubes

Blend on high for 60 - 90 seconds. *You can replace the greens with a quality green-drink extract like Organifi. Serves 2.

4. Banana Ginger Smoothie - Great for a snack or anytime you are having digestive issues. Soothes stomach trouble using fresh ginger, nut milk, and cinnamon.

1 large banana
10 oz almond or soy milk
1/2 tablespoon honey or maple syrup
1/2 teaspoon of cinnamon
2 ice cubes
1 thumb sized portion of ginger root

Blend on high for 60 - 90 seconds. Serve immediately.

5. Berry Vanilla Smoothie - This tangy smoothie is antioxidant-rich, and great way to get your Vitamin C.

1 cup strawberries
1 cup blueberries, blackberries, or raspberries
1/2 cup spinach
1 cup vanilla unsweetened almond or soy milk
1/2 cup pineapple
1 tablespoon vanilla protein powder

Blend on high for 60 - 90 seconds. *You can replace the spinach with a quality green-drink extract like Organifi. Serves 2.

What Is Juicing?

When we talk about juicing, we mean drinking **fresh-pressed or squeezed, mostly vegetable juice**. Canned or packaged fruit juices don't count, and neither does Jamba Juice or any of the big juice brands like Naked Juice (owned by Pepsi), or Odwalla (owned by Coca-Cola).

Many of those are not fresh (which means they have to add preservatives), and all of them are literally full of sugar without the fiber, which is why they tend to taste so good, because they are addictive like candy.

I recommend juicing with fresh veggies like celery, kale, carrots, cucumbers, and beets which have a rapid absorption of minerals and nutrients into your body. You can add fruits, but keep the ration 3 to 1 (in other words, 75% veggies)

If you have never juiced before, there's a movie called *Fat, Sick, and Nearly Dead* you can watch for free online. It's a great introduction to the topic.

Many towns have fresh juice bars these days, so feel free to let someone else do the hard work (and clean up too). Of course, that can get expensive, and if you want to save some money, I recommend you get a juicer.

I got my first one at a garage sale for $10 and it literally changed my life. You really don't have to spend a bunch of money. I highly recommend picking up a copy of *The Juicing Bible by Pat Crocker*.

It explains how to choose a juicing machine, how to use it for maximum efficiency, and contains hundreds of juicing recipes listed by the health condition you are trying to treat.

And remember, you can juice any vegetables or fruits you like! There are no rules in juicing. As long as you are getting the foods on the shopping list into your body, it doesn't matter how you mix and match them when you prepare fresh juice.

Here are a few of my favorite juicing recipes…

1. Morning Sunshine - This is my favorite, I try to have it once a week, and daily when I'm cleansing.

- 1 green apple
- 5 stalks of celery, leaves removed
- 1/2 cucumber
- 5 or 6 kale leaves
- 1/2 lemon, peeled
- 1 thumb sized portion of ginger root
- 1 thumb sized portion of turmeric root
- 1/2 cup cilantro

2. Liver Lover's Tonic - This is for anytime you want to support your liver and encourage liver healing.

- 2 cups purple cabbage
- 6 stalks of celery, leaves removed
- 1/2 green apple
- 1/2 cup of dandelion greens
- 3" - 4" of burdock root
- 1 thumb sized portion of turmeric root
- 1/2 cup cilantro

3. Purple and Orange - This is primarily made from root vegetables, which help you relax and ground you emotionally. It should be consumed towards the end of the day.

- 2 large red beets
- 6 carrots
- 2 cloves of garlic
- 1 thumb sized portion of ginger root
- 3" - 4" of burdock root

4. Green Machine - This supports proper digestion and healthy, regular bowel movements. I usually drink this during the liquid part of the cleanse since it has a tendency to "clean you out."

- 1/2 bunch of spinach, with stalks
- 6 stalks of celery, leaves removed
- 1/2 bunch of watercress, with stalks
- 1" - 2" of aloe vera
- 4 leaves Swiss chard
- 1/2 green apple

CHAPTER 18
Healthy Liver Shopping List

We mentioned earlier that healthy eating starts with a good, well-written shopping list. Here's a starting point for making your own grocery list that will encourage the consumption of liver-loving foods.

Always remember that organic foods and produce are best. Not only do they have fewer pesticides, herbicides, and other chemical compounds, but they may even be more nutritious. Of course, a non-organic apple is going to be better for you than an organic candy bar, but I think you see my point.

You may notice some foods appear multiple times on this list. That is because they qualify as multiple types of foods. Foods are listed by group (vegetables, fruits, etc.) for quick and easy reference and shopping.

...tables

- Broccoli
- Broccolini
- Bok choy
- Cauliflower
- Brussel sprouts
- Collard greens
- Mustard greens
- Turnip greens
- Spinach
- Bibb lettuce
- Romaine lettuce
- Chard
- Arugula
- Celery
- Kale
- Cabbage
- Napa cabbage
- Spinach
- Cucumbers
- Tomatoes
- Carrots
- Celery
- Avocados
- Fennel
- Beets
- Cucumber
- Zucchini
- Artichokes
- Asparagus
- Olives

Berries

- Strawberries
- Blueberries
- Raspberries
- Blackberries
- Acai berries
- Cranberries
- Salmonberries
- Boysenberries
- Ollalieberries

Fruits

- Goji berries
- Grapefruits
- Lemons and limes
- Oranges
- Papaya
- Bananas
- Apples
- Watermelon
- Cantaloupe
- Acerola cherries

Sweeteners

- Honey
- Coconut sugar
- Stevia
- Maple Syrup

Legumes

- Kidney beans
- Black beans
- Navy beans
- Mung Beans
- Chickpeas
- Lentils
- Split peas

Sprouts

- Alfalfa
- Sunflower
- Mung bean
- Wheat grass
- Barley grass

Herbs

- Milk thistle
- Turmeric
- Dandelion
- Burdock Root
- Artichoke
- Ginger root

Whole grains

- Quinoa
- Brown Rice
- Oatmeal
- Farro
- Barley
- Sprouted Tortillas
- Brown Rice Tortillas
- Wild Rice
- Millet

Fats

- Walnut oil
- Olive oil
- Avocado oil
- Flaxseed oil
- Hemp oil

Nuts

- Almonds
- Almond butter
- Macadamia nuts
- Walnuts
- Hazelnuts
- Brazil nuts

Seeds

- Pumpkin seeds
- Sunflower seeds
- Flaxseeds

PART IV: FATTY LIVER CLEANSE

CHAPTER 19

The Truth About Cleansing

You now know which foods to eat and which to avoid for a healthy liver, and you have a basic diet plan to follow.

You realize there are environmental factors that may be harming your liver, and understand the importance of keeping your home, workplace, body, and mind free of toxins.

Finally, you get how physical movement can have a positive effect on your liver health, and why your mindset may be a critical part of living a fulfilled and happy life.

In this next section, we will look at exactly how I cleaned up my own liver in a short period of time through cleansing. You can follow my lead, and hopefully, reverse the damage and begin the cellular regeneration process yourself.

What Exactly Is A Liver Cleanse?

The term liver cleanse means different things to different people, so let's get clear about when we are referring to here.

As you know, the liver filters the blood in your body and is a principal player in the breakdown of fat and the production of hormones. When we say liver cleanse, we are talking about consuming an **extremely clean, heavily liquid diet** for a short period of time (usually about a week).

A cleanse helps your liver get healthy by feeding it exactly what it needs, while at the same time, removing environmental and food-based toxins from your diet and environment that harm liver function.

Personally, I cleanse twice a year (in the spring and fall) and recommend you do the same. However, if you haven't ever done a cleanse, I recommend you begin at least **30 days after** you have followed the Fatty Liver Diet and gotten your body prepared.

Even if you have an otherwise normal liver, a cleanse takes quite a bit of "load" off your body, removing poisons, chemicals, heavy metals, and establishing good dietary practices and habits. It promotes oxygenation, alkalinity, and for me is like hitting a reset button on all my organs.

Still, it's something you want to ease into gently.

How Does a Cleanse Work?

Your liver is going 24 hours a day, 7 days a week, whether you are sleeping or awake, working, at home, playing, or on vacation. It is constantly filtering your blood, turning red blood cells into bile, aiding digestion, regulating hormones, and removing anything it deems a threat.

By eliminating both food-based and environmental toxins from your life, while **simultaneously** consuming things that support it, the liver should be able to direct it's energy to regeneration and healing itself.

I can only speak for myself, but my first cleanse got me to a place that shocked my doctor (in a good way). After 3 months on the Fatty Liver Diet and a 7 day cleanse, my enzyme numbers returned to normal, my skin cleared up, my attitude got better, and I lost my first 20 lbs. (This is not an exaggeration… I had to buy new clothes because the old ones were too loose.)

After another 2 months on the diet, I was down another 10 lbs, and all my blood work was back to normal. I was able to sleep again and had more energy while awake. Even better, my doctor **could not find evidence** that I even had fatty liver anymore.

Of course, everyone is different. You must always listen to your body and your doctor. If you are experiencing difficulties, ease up. Enjoying a longer and more gradual cleanse is better than trying to get it over and done with.

How to Cleanse Your Liver

There are eight specific steps that make up a healthy liver cleanse.

1 – Remove Toxicity: Remove all foods (and non-food items) from the "things your liver hates" section of this program. If you were cheating before, do NOT cheat during this phase of the process. In other words, no refined sugar or processed food of any kind. No white bread, biscuits, cakes or other baked goods. No meat or animal products. Replace dairy with nut milk, and of course, don't use cigarettes, drugs, or alcohol.

2 – Eat Clean With A Focus On Whole Food Plant Based Meals: As always, opt for fresh, organic foods whenever you can. Replace toxic food with the foods in the Diet Section and you will find yourself feeling full and satisfied. Get your daily protein from non-meat sources like legumes, beans, veggies, and nuts. Eat plenty of leafy greens, as well as anti-oxidant foods like citrus, asparagus, beets, and carrots.

3 – Supplement The Process: Earlier, we discussed adding supplements to a normal, daily, liver-loving diet. When I cleanse, I take probiotics, digestive enzymes, and liver boosting supplements like B-Max, milk thistle, dandelion root, vitamin E, vitamin C, and turmeric. While I don't recommend every supplement on a regular basis, I do find they are beneficial during my cleanse.

4 – Water and Lemon: Each morning, before I eat or drink anything, I add the juice from 1/2 of a lemon to 16 oz of pure, filtered, warm water. I drink this as soon as I wake up. Your body has been going through a natural filtration process while you sleep. This lemon/water mixture cranks up that process and activates your liver. Try to drink this healthy concoction over 15 - 20 minutes: It should be sipped, not gulped.

5 – Hydration: In addition to lemon water, there are several other things you should be drinking throughout the day during your cleanse to encourage the flushing out of toxins; Water, herbal tea, green tea, green drinks, smoothies, and freshly made organic vegetable juices. As we discovered after the disaster in Detroit, tap water can contain dangerous toxins and may be unsafe depending on where you live. We recommend you buy and use a water filter like the ZERO that reduces lead and other pollutants. Also, get yourself a large glass or Mason Jar and sip several times an hour instead of drinking large quantities all at once. Constantly giving your body water or other liquids helps your liver clean itself out. Not to mention it makes you feel full so you won't want to eat as much. A lot of the time we think we are hungry when we are really just dehydrated.

6 – Movement: You should normally get 90 minutes of movement daily, but that may be difficult while you are cleansing because you might be more tired than normal. If that seems like too much, you can cut this down to 20 - 30 minutes and engage in moderate activity, like walking or swimming. The amount of time you spend is more important than what you do, just try to keep moving.

7 – Detox Your Mind: You should always stay away from toxic people and environments, but when you are cleansing, it's extra important because you may be weaker or more susceptible to outside influences. By all means, take a break from the news, social media, or any situation, place, or person that makes you tense. Try to meditate each day, preferably in the morning, if only for a few minutes.

This 7 step liver cleanse process will dramatically help detox your body. It gives your liver a rest and allows it to naturally rebuild itself. I also usually allocate a few days In the middle of my liver cleanse for a *liquid-only* part.

The Power Of Liquids

During the cleanse, you **are** allowed to eat food, but you mostly want to focus on liquids like water, tea, green drinks, smoothies, and freshly made juice. I'll give you the actual schedule I follow in a bit, but you will probably find drinking liquids easier to handle if you ease into it.

Feel free to modify the schedule or the cleanse as you see fit. You can make it longer, shorter, or even eliminate it if you want. Remember you are the boss.

If you have never done a liquid diet, the most difficult part is the mental aspect. You've been eating all your life, and as we discussed previously, you likely have a strong connection to food.

Unfortunately, most people eat way more than they drink. They don't get enough hydration or healthy liquids into their bodies, and the liquids they do get (like soda-pop) are devoid of nutrition.

This is one of the big reasons we have liver problems. Your liver needs lots and lots of liquid to do its job properly and naturally keep itself clean. Take your weight, divide it by 3, and that's how many ounces of liquid you should be drinking a day under normal circumstances.

So for example, if you weigh 150 pounds, you should be drinking 50 ounces at a minimum, or 4 - 7 cups a day for women, and 6 - 11 cups a day for men.

Bathroom Break

A 12-ounce smoothie you make fresh from organic fruits, vegetables, roots, and herbs floods your system with a lot of liquid food. As part of the detoxing process, you may find yourself expelling a lot of waste material, and sometimes having the urge to do so quickly.

It's not uncommon needing to use the restroom every few hours. This is **good**. It's a sign your body is getting rid of toxins and poisons that are causing health problems, and your digestive tract is cleaning itself up.

During the liquid part of the cleanse, you want to drink one large smoothie or juice at breakfast, one at lunch, and one at dinner. Throughout the day, keep yourself hydrated.

If you do not have organic vegetables and fruits, get the freshest produce you can, look online for farmers markets and farm stands near you.

And make sure to clean your produce completely, regardless of whether it's organic or conventional. Mix a tablespoon of salt and some apple cider vinegar in a spray bottle and fill with water to spray on your food to clean off contaminants, and if needed, scrub produce with a soft vegetable brush.

Make This Plan Work for You, Not Against You

These different behaviors may be hard to adopt because they are so foreign to what you have been doing your entire life.

However, your body is in a state of disrepair. I know how it feels. I had to change many negative behaviors I had been doing all my whole life, and which led to my health problems, and it was tough at first.

These new habits, like drinking a lot of liquids, are likely going to deliver benefits you have not previously enjoyed. They'll probably make you feel younger and more vibrant, and are definitely good news for your liver.

CHAPTER 20

Setting Your Intention

Before you cleanse, there is something to think about…

Why Are You Doing It?

That may sound like a silly question. Of course, you want to improve your health and well-being, and hopefully, flush the toxins from your body, maybe even lose a few pounds.

But you may also want to use this as an opportunity to **shift your habits** and establish new ones after your cleanse is over.

Are you going to return to your former lifestyle, eating things that harm your body and liver? Or are you going to take this wonderful opportunity to make nutrition, movement, and optimal health your new way of being?

You are going to feel great after you start the Fatty Liver Diet, and even more so after the cleanse. Many people notice they sleep better, feel better, their mind becomes sharp, and they don't experience as many ups and downs emotionally.

Some discover they have more energy than they have had in years. This is a common occurrence when you rid your body of toxins and get your organs healthy again.

When you feel that great, and have maybe even lost some weight, you might think you can go back to eating anything you like. After all, your system has been cleansed, you look and feel awesome, so why not reward yourself with some of your favorite foods that just happen to be unhealthy?

This dangerous thinking is why you need to consider your goals now, **before** you go through your cleanse. Set the intention for what you are doing and how you are going to move forward in the future.

One way to do that is with daily affirmations.

Honestly, these should be a part of your everyday life, not just during your cleanse. Affirmations have the power to focus your mind and keep you on the right track health-wise. They remind you of your "why" and the benefits of adopting a healthy lifestyle.

What Is an Affirmation?

One of my spiritual friends says that an affirmation is something you say to yourself that isn't true... yet. 😄

It's part visualization, part positive thinking, and part goal-setting. The most basic affirmations are statements which begin with the words "I am ... ".

- I am healthy.
- I am skinny.
- I am intelligent.
- I am loved.
- I am beautiful.
- I am powerful.

Pay attention to the wording. You don't say, "I <u>want</u> to be healthy" or "I <u>want</u> to lose weight" or "I <u>want</u> to be smart." You need to put your affirmations in the present tense.

By saying, "I am healthy" (even if you have not reached optimal health yet), your subconscious begins to think healthy thoughts and you make **smarter food and lifestyle choices** rather than opting for actions that could harm your body. This also creates a situation in your mind called **cognitive dissonance**, which means there's a difference between the way things are and the way you are affirming them.

See, if your mind says "I am healthy" but your body says "I am sick," one or the other will need to come into alignment, and if you regularly say "I am healthy," it sends a message to your brain, which **sends a message back to your body to get with the program**.

Always write your affirmations as *positives*. Instead of saying, "I am not addicted to alcohol," say "I am alcohol-free." You see how much better that sounds? Here are a few of my affirmations…

- I love my liver.
- My liver is healthy and vibrant.
- I am in excellent health.
- I lovingly forgive and release all the past.
- I choose to fill my life with joy.
- I love and approve of myself.
- I create my own reality.
- My health is excellent.
- The foods I eat make me healthy.
- My mind is clear and focused.

- I am in control of my emotions.
- I am growing stronger and healthier each day.
- I am attracted to healthy people and situations.

Feel free to use these as is, or as guidelines to brainstorm your own affirmations. Try to keep them short, repeat them several times each morning, and before you go to bed. You might also want to write them out in a notebook.

They may seem simplistic, and they are. But their power cannot be overstated, because when you tell yourself something over and over, it gets your subconscious working on creating that reality behind-the-scenes, almost like magic.

As personal development expert Earl Nightingale was fond of saying, "We become what we think about."

CHAPTER 21
Preparing For Your Cleanse

Your mind craves order. When you do specific things at the same time every day, your brain notices this pattern. Conscious effort becomes unconscious habit.

Have you ever heard of an athlete getting "psyched up" before a big game or competition? This is a process where they prepare themselves mentally for what is about to happen.

If they didn't do this, and simply waited until the game began without thinking about who they are playing or how to prepare, their performance would most definitely suffer.

You will benefit from the same type of mental preparation when you are getting ready for your liver cleanse.

What do you need to think about when you are starting?

You should remember the cleansing process can be **traumatic** to your body because of the built up fat. and toxins stored in that fat. Your emotions, hormones, energy levels and other physical or mental factors may also be affected: You could experience emotional ups and downs, and possibly weakness or fatigue, both mentally and physically.

Your stress hormones are going to be triggered because your body will see your cleanse as an attack of sorts. So cortisol can spike from time to time, and that means you could be edgy, intense, with all of your senses preparing for what they perceive as a threat.

Knowing this beforehand, if you see anger or frustration which doesn't seem to have any cause, it's probably the cleanse your body is going through. Take a few minutes to find a quiet spot and clear your mind. Have a conversation with yourself, and remember this is a process you will benefit from in many ways.

Most people get through their cleanse just fine, with only minimal disturbances.

However, some take time off work due to the lack of energy they feel. You may decide to take a full 7 days off so the emotional highs and lows don't affect your performance, especially if you do physical labor.

Just remember, you are doing your cleanse for a very good reason ... to thank your liver for all the hard work it does, and to become healthier in body and mind. Congratulate yourself for taking personal responsibility for your health, even if that means a little discomfort.

It's only 7 days, you can get through this.

CHAPTER 22

Your Morning Ritual

Science has shown that human beings get better at activities the more they repeat them. If they repeat every day, at around the same time, those activities become what is known as **habits**.

As your brain gets used to a new habit, it starts to prepare ahead of time and often "clears the way" so the habit can naturally progress. So for example, if you set your alarm for 6:45 AM every morning as part of your cleanse process, after about a month, you will probably start waking up on your own.

Even more interesting, your brain tells the rest of your body that your morning ritual is about to begin, and you start to look forward to getting out of bed.

I recommend you begin what I call a morning ritual, which is an easy, productive, fun way to prepare for your day. Here is a short list of things you may want to include. I have found the following things never fail to get me started each day on the right foot.

Add your own ideas. Make your morning ritual your own.

Think positive thoughts - Each morning, before you even get out of bed, tell yourself that today is going to be wonderfully rewarding and that you are going to sail over any speed bumps or hurdles with no problems.

Be loving - If you are in a relationship, lean over and tell your partner that you love them, and give them a little kiss. That's a great way for both of you to begin each day, feeling loved and supported.

Start with affirmations - Positive statements can have a dramatic impact on creating the destiny you desire, or at the least, helping you begin on the right foot.

Lemon Water- As I mentioned before, I combine 16 ounces of pure, filtered warm water with the juice from 1/2 a lemon so I'm fully hydrated before I eat, start moving, or drink anything that has caffeine.

Breathe - Breathing exercises fill your lungs with healthy oxygen, clear your mind and help you relax and focus. This is a great way to start your day. There are some excellent breathing tips and practices proven to help you de-stress and clear your mind in the index.

The following books do a great job of helping you to guide and control your thoughts. I highly recommend them as a way to expand your consciousness, as well as to support a healthy morning ritual.

- o *The Morning Miracle* - Hal Elrod

- o *The Power of Now*: A Guide to Spiritual Enlightenment - Eckhart Tolle

- o *Every Day Tao*: Self-Help in the Here and Now - Leonard Willoughby

- o *Change Your Thoughts, Change Your Life*: Living the Wisdom of the Tao - Dr. Wayne W. Dyer

It doesn't matter which religion or spiritual practice you follow, these books will help you become more mindful and make your life easier.

CHAPTER 23

Making a Schedule

Some people like fixed schedules that are easy to follow. Others like to be given the facts so they can create their own process.

One of the great things about this program is that it's very flexible. You can take the information you have been given, and create a plan that fits your unique situation. Or you can just follow my *personal* step-by-step cleanse schedule, that is easy to follow, and fully adaptable.

For People Who Want to Create Their Own Schedule

You have all the information you need to enjoy a healthy liver cleanse and establish good health habits going forward. Simply stick to the foods and drinks listed in the Fatty Liver Diet for 3 weeks before and after your cleanse.

You may include some of the things your liver loves (Chapter 10), just so long as you avoid foods and activities your liver hates (Chapter 9).

During your cleanse, cut your movement to 20 - 30 minutes a day, and remember to only eat when you are hungry, aiming for 3 main meals each day, as well as 2 - 3 snacks.

After you are done with the cleanse, you can continue to enjoy a healthy liver and overall wellness like I do by following the Fatty Liver Diet and daily movement on a regular basis.

For People Who Want A Ready-Made Schedule

For me, the hardest part of cleansing is organizing everything so I'll be able to actually follow through. That's why I came up with a simple schedule that outlines my meals and daily activity in detail.

I always begin with the Fatty Liver Diet, and try to stay on that for at least a month so I can **transition** into the cleanse slowly. I also begin my supplement regimen about a week beforehand. The goal is to prepare my body and mind for the healing process that will follow. The schedule looks like this...

- Days 1 - 21 - Begin the Fatty Liver Diet, which is whole food and plant based. If you were already on the diet but were cheating every now and then, begin following it to the letter.

- Days 22 - 28 - Continue with diet, add probiotics, B-Max, Vitamin E and C, Milk Thistle, and digestive enzymes.

- Days 29 - 33 - Begin cleanse, following the program laid out later in this chapter.

- Days 34 - 35 - Liquids only for 2 days. Juice and blend healthy vegetables and fruits, and drink plenty of water. You may enjoy Miso soup, and if you are feeling very hungry, have a bowl of vegetable soup.

- Days 36 - 42 - Stop supplements except for probiotic, and go back to Fatty Liver Diet.

Making the cleanse your own will give you the best chance at success. No one knows your body as well as you do, but remember, challenging yourself a little will have great rewards also.

CHAPTER 24

My 7-Day Liver Cleanse

The liver cleanse itself lasts 7 days, but you can see from the schedule in the previous chapter that there are actually **42 days** in the whole process. That's because you want to ease into it gradually, and ease out when you are done.

Cleanses can be difficult if you regularly eat junk food, or sugar, or a lot of simple carbohydrates, and you may even experience withdrawal symptoms. Not surprising considering that a recent study showed sugar is more addictive than cocaine.

The physical and mental effects food has on us are significant, and shouldn't be underestimated. If you ever feel a particular emotion when you eat a certain kind of food, it's probably because of an association you have from your past.

While many memories are good, some, like feelings of loneliness, emptiness, or sadness can be deadly, tricking us into eating things that harm our bodies to satisfy an emotional need. If that sounds uncomfortably familiar, just know I'm right there with you. I had all those food associations too, and they almost killed me…

But they didn't!

So let's get down to the brass tacks. Even though this cleanse is technically just for a week, expect unfamiliar feelings to emerge. Avoiding foods you have been eating your whole life, and possibly eating some foods you aren't familiar with can be difficult.

I get it, that's why they call it "comfort" food. Just remember that it's **not** comfortable to your body or health, and it's definitely not comfortable to your liver.

If you feel yourself slipping, **just remember most people can do anything for one week.** The physical and mental pain of having a compromised liver is far worse than stepping out of your food "comfort" zone.

You deserve to reclaim your life and get your health back on track.

Say your affirmations, do your breathing exercises, get plenty of sleep, keep hydrated, stay away from negative situations and people, give yourself a chance to get healthy, and get your strength back.

The simple fact that you bought this program, and started your healthy liver quest means you are **on your way** to greater awareness and attention to your liver, and that's a wonderful first step.

Learn To Identify Genuine Hunger

Some people think that cleanses are about starving yourself, but I disagree. A properly designed cleanse will rarely leave you feeling hungry. You should actually feel <u>less</u> hungry because you'll be fully hydrated, well nourished, and quite satisfied.

Not to mention your stomach will start to shrink, and you may find yourself needing less food than you normally do. That's another benefit of this program, you won't been eating as much as you were before, and what you are eating is going to be substantially better for you.

In fact, if you avoid sugar, alcohol, and simple carbohydrates, your food cravings will start to diminish. After a month on the diet, they'll actually begin to disappear. Pay attention to what you put into your mouth and try to eat slower. Most of us eat very quickly, and that doesn't give our brains enough time to catch up with our stomach.

About halfway through every meal, take a short break, relax, and breathe for a few minutes. You may find your stomach is actually **full** before you are finished with your serving. At that point, stop! There's nothing wrong with having leftovers, especially if it keeps you from overeating.

Salt and Sodium

There's strong evidence that salt intake is hard on your liver due to increased blood pressure and hypertension it causes. Not to mention it can lead to abdominal pain, tenderness, and in some cases, even nausea.

I recommend eliminating table salt from your diet completely. If you use salt, make it sea-salt or a product like *Braggs*, and keep all sodium-based enhancers to a minimum. The good news is as you clean up your diet, you may find yourself needing less and less salt with your food because your taste buds return to enjoying natural un-salted flavors.

Colonics And Enemas

It's optional but highly recommended that during the cleanse, you give yourself a warm-water enema every other day to help clean your bowels and clear out any toxins or undigested food still in your body.

Even better, find a professional colonic therapist, and plan to have a colonic a day or two after your cleanse. It's amazing what they can remove and how much better you'll feel when you are completely clean on the inside. Last time I had a colonic, I lost 3 pounds of pure junk that was slowing me down and making me heavy and bloated.

Getting Everyone In Your House On The Cleanse Program

One of the hardest things about cleansing is not what you can and can't eat, but what other people are eating around you. If you are making Mac and Cheese for your kids, or a steak for your spouse, or if your roommate comes home with a large pizza, it's going to be a **lot harder** to focus on staying healthy.

Whenever I cleanse, I let my friends family know I'm going to need their support. I try to engineer situations where I'll have a good chance of success, which means planning things out beforehand. For example, I make things for dinner I know my wife will like too (stirfrys, salads, veggie chili, etc.).

Sometimes she's open to doing the cleanse with me, but if not, that's OK. My cleanse is about me and making my body healthy. If she's hankering for a burger, she'll usually go out with a friend so I don't have to cook it for her (along with my own meal).

Other people in your household don't need to cleanse with you, but they do need to support you by not offering you food (or buying food) you are actively trying to avoid. If you are an ice-cream addict, the easiest way to win the healthy eating game is to not have ice-cream in the house to begin with.

And while we are on the topic, the easiest way to cleanse is to have a fridge full of fresh juices and veggies. Chop up some carrots and celery, and stick them in a bowl in the front part of your refrigerator. Then, when you get hungry and you're on the prowl for something to eat, you are presented with a healthy snack, conveniently cut up into bite-sized pieces.

A kitchen filled with veggies and fruits and beans and nuts and legumes and other good stuff means that "healthy" becomes the default, which is where you want to eventually get to in order to save your liver.

On to the cleanse…

Day 1 and 2 - Fatty Liver Cleanse

Day one is usually not that hard for me because I have been on the Fatty Liver Diet for a month, my body has already gone through whatever withdrawals it needs to go through (from eliminating sugar and carbs). Day two gets a little more difficult, but a lot of it is psychological.

Morning lemon and water - Add the juice from one half of a fresh lemon into 16 ounces of warm water. Drink first thing in the morning and take your probiotic supplement, before breakfast. I like to do my breathing exercises in between my lemon water and green tea.

Breakfast – Choose one of the following:

- A fresh fruit salad (papaya, banana, berries,) topped with 2 tablespoons of hemp seeds, chopped almonds, ground flaxseed or chia seeds.

- A 16 oz smoothie, with organic papaya, berries, half a banana, half cup of unsweetened nut milk and 2 ice cubes.

- A 16 oz Morning Sunshine juice.

- Small bowl of oatmeal with fruit and nut milk.

Mid-day snack – Choose one of the following:

- 1 sprouted tortilla with sliced bananas and almond butter. Or hummus, sliced avocado or organic guacamole.

- A 12 oz Morning Sunshine juice.

- A 12 oz Liver Lover's Tonic.

- One green or Fuji apple.

Lunch – Choose one of the following:

- A large salad with fresh greens, mixed veggies, and almonds or walnuts, drizzled with organic coconut oil, extra-virgin olive oil, fresh lemon juice and/or raw, unfiltered apple cider vinegar.

- Spread hummus or avocado (or both) on large washed romaine lettuce leaves, kale or collard greens. Add finely grated carrots, zucchini, beets, tomato, sunflower sprouts, and/or fresh green herbs. Wrap and enjoy.

- Make a healthy wrap with a sprouted tortilla. Use coconut oil, extra-virgin olive oil, hummus or guacamole in the place of mayonnaise. Layer your favorite greens with cucumber slices, tomatoes, portobello mushrooms, onions, or any other healthy vegetables.

- One small bowl of cooked brown rice with diced organic veggies, black beans, any herbs and spices you enjoy, drizzled with a little coconut oil or extra-virgin olive oil.

Afternoon snack – Choose one of the following:

- A 12 oz Liver Lover's Tonic.

- A 12 oz Purple and Orange juice.

- 2 - 3 celery sticks with almond butter.

Dinner – Choose one of the following:

- A large salad consisting mostly of fresh, raw, organic vegetables and leafy greens, your choice. You can sauté the veggies beforehand and eat them cold. Add a small handful of nuts such as walnuts, pine nuts or almonds.

- Veggie stirfry with any (or all) of the following: Carrots, beets, broccoli, string beans, asparagus, cauliflower, kale, peppers, onion. Serve over quinoa or brown rice and top with fresh herbs and spices.

- A medium sized bowl of veggie chili, with 1/2 cup of quinoa or brown rice.

- Brush large portobello mushroom caps with extra-virgin olive oil or organic coconut oil and roast for 10 - 15 minutes. Use these caps in place of bread, making healthy sandwiches with avocado, hummus, or well as your favorite vegetables.

- A 16 oz Purple and Orange juice.

Evening snack - Only eat if you are hungry

- A 12 oz Purple and Orange juice.

- 1 oz raw cacao nibs.

Day 3 - Fatty Liver Cleanse

Day three is a bit more focused on juicing. This is traditionally the hardest day for me. I try to take time off from work and plan to spend time in nature, and away from media, Facebook, and any negative situations (or people).

Morning lemon and water - Add the juice from one half of a fresh lemon into 16 ounces of warm water. Drink first thing in the morning and take your probiotic supplement, before breakfast. I like to do my breathing exercises in between my lemon water and green tea.

Breakfast – Choose one of the following:

- A fresh fruit salad (papaya, banana, berries,) topped with 2 tablespoons of hemp seeds, chopped almonds, ground flaxseed or chia seeds.

- A 16 oz smoothie, with organic papaya, berries, half a banana, half cup of unsweetened nut milk and 2 ice cubes.

- A 20 oz Morning Sunshine juice.

Mid-day snack – Choose one of the following:

- 1 sprouted tortilla with sliced bananas, hummus, sliced avocado or organic guacamole.

- A 12 oz Morning Sunshine juice.

- A 12 oz Liver Lover's Tonic.

- One green or Fuji apple.

Lunch – Choose one of the following:

- A large salad with fresh greens, mixed veggies, and almonds or walnuts, drizzled with organic coconut oil, extra-virgin olive oil, fresh lemon juice and/or raw, unfiltered apple cider vinegar.

- Spread hummus or avocado (or both) on large washed romaine lettuce leaves, kale or collard greens. Add finely grated carrots, zucchini, beets, tomato, sunflower sprouts, and/or fresh green herbs. Wrap and enjoy.
- A 16 Liver Lover's Tonic.

- One small bowl of cooked brown rice with diced organic veggies, black beans, any herbs and spices you enjoy, drizzled with a little coconut oil or extra-virgin olive oil.

Afternoon snack – Choose one of the following:

- 2 oz of raw almonds.

- A 12 oz Liver Lover's Tonic.

- A 12 oz Purple and Orange juice.

- 2 - 3 celery sticks with almond butter.

Dinner – Choose one of the following:

- A large salad consisting mostly of fresh, raw, organic vegetables and leafy greens, your choice. You can salute the veggies beforehand and eat them cold. Add a small handful of nuts such as walnuts, pine nuts or almonds.

- Veggie stirfry with any (or all) of the following: Carrots, beets, broccoli, string beans, asparagus, cauliflower, kale, peppers, onion. Serve over quinoa or brown rice and top with fresh herbs and spices.

- A medium sized bowl of veggie chili, with 1/2 cup of quinoa or brown rice.

- Brush large portobello mushroom caps with extra-virgin olive oil or organic coconut oil. Use these caps in place of bread, making healthy sandwiches with avocado, hummus, or well as your favorite vegetables.

- A 16 oz Purple and Orange juice.

Evening snack - Only eat if you are hungry

- A 12 oz Purple and Orange juice.

- A 12 oz Green Monster juice.

- 1 oz raw cacao nibs.

Day 4 - Fatty Liver Cleanse (Liquids)

Day four is the first day of liquid only. My goal is to have 4 - 6 freshly prepared juices per day. Remember, you don't have to do this part if you don't want to, everything is optional. Listen to your body and if you feel like you need to eat, have a salad or bowl of soup, or just go back to the normal cleanse.

For me, the liquid-only part is pretty easy since I have usually started to see some real benefits, like deeper sleep, less joint pain, and weight loss. Once you see results, it's a lot easier to keep going.

From a logistical standpoint, I *always* plan my liquid-only part over a long weekend. The last thing I want to do is work while I'm not eating solids. Liquid-only days are nature days, I stay off the Internet, and usually take the time to read a book after a day hiking, or at the beach, or just spending time in nature.

Morning lemon and water - Add the juice from one half of a fresh lemon into 16 ounces of warm water. Drink first thing in the morning and take your probiotic supplement, before breakfast. I like to do my breathing exercises in between my lemon water and green tea.

Breakfast – Choose one of the following:

- A 16 oz smoothie, with organic papaya, berries, half a banana, half cup of unsweetened nut milk and 2 ice cubes.

- A 20 oz Morning Sunshine juice.

- A 20 oz Liver Lover's Tonic.

Mid-day snack – Choose one of the following:

- A 12 oz Morning Sunshine juice.

- A 12 oz Liver Lover's Tonic.

Lunch – Choose one of the following:

- A 16 oz smoothie, with organic papaya, berries, half a banana, half cup of unsweetened nut milk and 2 ice cubes.

- A 20 oz Morning Sunshine juice.

- A 20 oz Liver Lover's Tonic.

- A 20 oz Purple and Orange juice.

- A cup of veggie chili.

Afternoon snack – Choose one of the following:

- A 12 oz Liver Lover's Tonic.

- A 12 oz Purple and Orange juice.

- 12 oz of bone or chicken broth.

- A 12 oz Miso Soup with dulse or other seaweed.

Dinner – Choose one of the following:

- A 14 oz Green Monster juice.

- A 20 oz Liver Lover's Tonic.

- A 20 oz Purple and Orange juice.

- A cup of veggie chili or soup.

Evening snack - Only eat if you are hungry

- A 12 oz Purple and Orange juice.

- A 12 oz Green Monster juice.

Day 5 - Fatty Liver Cleanse (Liquids)

Day five is big, it's my <u>final</u> day of liquid only, and also when I take an afternoon oil-citrus mixture to clear out my liver and gallbladder (instructions are below).

When you do this, you might find that you need to go to the bathroom frequently, so definitely don't plan anything that afternoon or evening. In fact, you really should take it easy on day 5. I usually don't 'eat' dinner after the liquid-only part because I'm not hungry.

Morning lemon and water - Add the juice from one half of a fresh lemon into 16 ounces of warm water. Drink first thing in the morning and take your probiotic supplement, before breakfast. I like to do my breathing exercises in between my lemon water and green tea.

Breakfast – Choose one of the following:

- A 16 oz smoothie, with organic papaya, berries, half a banana, half cup of unsweetened nut milk and 2 ice cubes.

- A 20 oz Morning Sunshine juice.

- A 20 oz Liver Lover's Tonic.

Mid-day snack – Choose one of the following:

- A 12 oz Morning Sunshine juice.

- A 12 oz Liver Lover's Tonic.

Lunch – Choose one of the following:

- A 16 oz smoothie, with organic papaya, berries, half a banana, half cup of unsweetened nut milk and 2 ice cubes.

- A 20 oz Morning Sunshine juice.

- A 20 oz Liver Lover's Tonic.

- A 20 oz Purple and Orange juice.

- A cup of veggie chili.

Afternoon snack – Do the following:

- Instead of an afternoon snack, mix 4 oz of organic olive oil with 4 oz of citrus juice like grapefruit or orange. Drink it all, and lay on your right side for 30 - 60 minutes. The mixture will activate your liver and gallbladder, causing toxins to be released during your next bowel movement.

Dinner – Choose one of the following:

- A 14 oz Green Monster juice.

- A 20 oz Liver Lover's Tonic.

- A cup of veggie chili.

Evening snack - Only eat if you are hungry

- A 12 oz Purple and Orange juice.

- A 12 oz Green Monster juice.

Day 6 - Fatty Liver Cleanse

Day six we go back to the normal cleanse, which is a lot easier since we can eat food again. I like to plan a colonic for this day, to help me get all the toxins and crap (literally) out of my body. You can, of course, do an enema on your own, but a colonic goes much deeper and cleans you out more effectively.

Morning lemon and water - Add the juice from one half of a fresh lemon into 16 ounces of warm water. Drink first thing in the morning and take your probiotic supplement, before breakfast. I like to do my breathing exercises in between my lemon water and green tea.

Breakfast – Choose 1 of the following:

- A fresh fruit salad (papaya, banana, berries,) topped with 2 tablespoons of hemp seeds, chopped almonds, ground flaxseed or chia seeds.

- A 16 oz smoothie, with organic papaya, berries, half a banana, half cup of unsweetened nut milk and 2 ice cubes.

- A 16 oz Morning Sunshine juice.

- Small bowl of oatmeal with fruit and nut milk.

Mid-day snack – Choose one of the following:

- 1 sprouted tortilla with sliced bananas, hummus, sliced avocado or organic guacamole.

- A 12 oz Morning Sunshine juice.

- A 12 oz Liver Lover's Tonic.

- One green or Fuji apple.

Lunch – Choose 1 of the following:

- A large salad with fresh greens, mixed veggies, and almonds or walnuts, drizzled with organic coconut oil, extra-virgin olive oil, fresh lemon juice and/or raw, unfiltered apple cider vinegar.

- Spread hummus or avocado (or both) on large washed romaine lettuce leaves, kale or collard greens. Add finely grated carrots, zucchini, beets, tomato, sunflower sprouts, and/or fresh green herbs. Wrap and enjoy.

- Make a healthy wrap with a sprouted tortilla. Use coconut oil, extra-virgin olive oil, hummus or guacamole in the place of mayonnaise. Layer your favorite greens with cucumber slices, tomatoes, portobello mushrooms, onions, or any other healthy vegetables.

- One small bowl of cooked brown rice with diced organic veggies, black beans, any herbs and spices you enjoy, drizzled with a little coconut oil or extra-virgin olive oil.

Afternoon snack – Choose one of the following:

- A 12 oz Liver Lover's Tonic.

- A 12 oz Purple and Orange juice.

- 2 - 3 celery sticks with almond butter.

Dinner – Choose one of the following:

- A large salad consisting mostly of fresh, raw, organic vegetables and leafy greens, your choice. You can sauté the veggies beforehand and eat them cold. Add a small handful of nuts such as walnuts, pine nuts or almonds.

- Veggie stirfry with any (or all) of the following: Carrots, beets, broccoli, string beans, asparagus, cauliflower, kale, peppers, onion, garlic, turmeric, ginger. Serve over quinoa or brown rice and top with fresh herbs and spices.

- A medium sized bowl of veggie chili, with 1/2 cup of quinoa or brown rice.

- Brush large portobello mushroom caps with extra-virgin olive oil or organic coconut oil. Use these caps in place of bread, making healthy sandwiches with avocado, hummus, or well as your favorite vegetables.

- A 16 oz Purple and Orange juice.

Evening snack - Only eat if you are hungry

- A 12 oz Purple and Orange juice.

- 1 oz raw cacao nibs.

Day 7 - Fatty Liver Cleanse

Last day of the cleanse (Yay!). By now, I'm feeling pretty good, and have started to see significant weight loss. My energy is up, and I no longer am up in a fog.

Morning lemon and water - Add the juice from one half of a fresh lemon into 16 ounces of warm water. Drink first thing in the morning and take your probiotic supplement, before breakfast. I like to do my breathing exercises in between my lemon water and green tea.

Breakfast – Choose 1 of the following:

- A fresh fruit salad (papaya, banana, berries,) topped with 2 tablespoons of hemp seeds, chopped almonds, ground flaxseed or chia seeds.

- A 16 oz smoothie, with organic papaya, berries, half a banana, half cup of unsweetened nut milk and 2 ice cubes.

- A 16 oz Morning Sunshine juice.

- Small bowl of oatmeal with fruit and nut milk.

Mid-day snack – Choose one of the following:

- 1 sprouted tortilla with sliced bananas, hummus, sliced avocado or organic guacamole.

- A 12 oz Morning Sunshine juice.

- A 12 oz Liver Lover's Tonic.

- One green or Fuji apple.

Lunch – Choose 1 of the following:

- A large salad with fresh greens, mixed veggies, and almonds or walnuts, drizzled with organic coconut oil, extra-virgin olive oil, fresh lemon juice and/or raw, unfiltered apple cider vinegar.

- Spread hummus or avocado (or both) on large washed romaine lettuce leaves, kale or collard greens. Add finely grated carrots, zucchini, beets, tomato, sunflower sprouts, and/or fresh green herbs. Wrap and enjoy.

- Make a healthy wrap with a sprouted tortilla. Use coconut oil, extra-virgin olive oil, hummus or guacamole in the place of mayonnaise. Layer your favorite greens with cucumber slices, tomatoes, portobello mushrooms, onions, or any other healthy vegetables.

- One small bowl of cooked brown rice with diced organic veggies, black beans, any herbs and spices you enjoy, drizzled with a little coconut oil or extra-virgin olive oil.

Afternoon snack – Choose one of the following:

- A 12 oz Liver Lover's Tonic.

- A 12 oz Purple and Orange juice.

- 2 - 3 celery sticks with almond butter.

Dinner – Choose one of the following:

- A large salad consisting mostly of fresh, raw, organic vegetables and leafy greens, your choice. You can sauté the veggies beforehand and eat them cold. Add a small handful of nuts such as walnuts, pine nuts or almonds.

- Veggie stirfry with any (or all) of the following: Carrots, beets, broccoli, string beans, asparagus, cauliflower, kale, peppers, onion. Serve over quinoa or brown rice and top with fresh herbs and spices.

- A medium sized bowl of veggie chili, with 1/2 cup of quinoa or brown rice.

- Brush large portobello mushroom caps with extra-virgin olive oil or avocado oil. Use these caps in place of bread, making healthy sandwiches with avocado, hummus, or well as your favorite vegetables.

- A 16 oz Purple and Orange juice.

Evening snack - Only eat if you are hungry

- A 12 oz Purple and Orange juice.

- 1 oz raw cacao nibs.

These meal plans are simple, but they work. They are exactly what I follow when I cleanse, and I have even integrated them into my daily life and diet.

If you are ready for vibrant health and a reversal of your liver issues, I invite you to give this food program a shot. You really have nothing to lose, and a much healthier liver to gain.

CHAPTER 25

Support And Enhance Your Cleanse

Let's take a look at a few other resources and practices that help you get the most out of your cleanse. Some of these techniques are new, and some have been used for hundreds of years, and are very effective for promoting liver health and healing.

- Join our **Fatty Liver Facebook Group** (see link in the back) or other online support forum. Facebook and other social media sites, as well as liver disease forums, put you in touch with others that have already done what you are about to undertake, and are in a great position to offer support.

- Find a buddy. Online support groups are great, but there is nothing like joining up a friend or family member in the pursuit of good health for support and motivation. Not to mention a buddy helps you become more accountable.

- Consider a colonic. Also called colonic hydrotherapy or colon irrigation, this is where you visit a spa or hydrotherapist and have them flush out your colon and remove the excess junk in there. I typically do this at the end of my cleanse, but you can consider it whenever you are feeling full or stuffed up. Bonus: you usually lose a few pounds after a colonic, and often times have a lot more energy.

- A good old-fashioned enema was the healing tool of choice for a number of gastrointestinal and liver conditions hundreds of years ago. It's easy and you can do it yourself. Warm spring water (around 95 degrees) is the safest and most comfortable.

- Massage, and specifically Chinese massage (also known as Chi New Tsang) stimulates the organs and colon, reviving them and helping to release toxins and fats. However, any massage will put you into a parasympathetic state, reduce pain, and lower your blood pressure.

- Epsom salt baths have been used for centuries as a powerful detoxing tool, and are quite inexpensive. These baths prevent magnesium deficiency, allowing you to more effectively fight inflammation and support healthy oxygenation throughout your body. This process also stimulates your digestive process and promotes healthy sleep while detoxing your body.

- Oil from the castor seed is used for a number of health treatments. Castor oil was used in ancient Japan, and can be found in both Ayurvedic and TCM practices. Rub castor oil on inflamed areas, and apply a heating pad or hot water bottle for a soothing way to reduce pain in liver and joints.

- The principal benefit of meditation is stress relief and a calm, focused mind. Even just 10 or 15 minutes of meditation daily can help you deal with the emotional ups and downs of liver issues.

- Yoga is thousands of years old. It has been used across multiple cultures to remove stress and anxiety, and certain yoga postures stimulate your liver to help you work more efficiently. Focus on these poses for maximum effect:

  o Big Toe Pose
  o Standing Forward Bend
  o Boat Pose
  o Cat Pose
  o Bridge Pose

What to Do When You Slip Up

If you fell out of a boat in shark infested waters, you would probably get back in pretty quickly, right?

Listen, humans are fallible. We all make mistakes, screw things up, fail to follow directions, and sometimes we even eat (or do) things that are bad for us. If you make a mistake or fall off the wagon, relax. The worst thing you can do is cause yourself a lot of unnecessary stress or grief.

Life happens. Sometimes you find yourself at an unhealthy restaurant when it's meal time. Sometimes there's a party at work, and you are handed a piece of cake. Sometimes you buy unhealthy food because you are rushing to get to work.

It's difficult to change lifelong behaviors, and that is exactly what I'm asking you to do, transform your life. Don't beat yourself up when you make mistakes. Instead, focus on congratulating yourself when you have small wins and learn to kick bad habits.

Set yourself up for success

Of all the things that helped me get healthy, the biggest one was planning ahead, and chances are, it will help you too:

- Find out where local farm-stands and farmers markets are located, and schedule time for your produce shopping. Often, the farmers will begin to recognize you as a regular shopper. This is a great moment to enjoy a new friendship based on good health.

- Make a detailed shopping list of healthy food you need for the week ahead, and avoid buying junk food or anything that's not good for you – that is, don't buy anything that didn't make the list. Remember, if it's not in your kitchen, you will be far less likely to eat it.

- Schedule time off from work during your cleanse. Don't cleanse around the holidays or other important celebrations. You may be anxious to get started right away, but blocking off time when you have few other obligations means a greater chance for success.

CHAPTER 26

What to Expect

Expect to be excited and motivated early on. Writing out your shopping list, visiting farmer's markets, creating delicious and nutritious meals, clearing old, unhealthy food out your pantry, these are all activities that will have you raring to go.

However, as you start living this new way, you may feel strange and unfamiliar emotions. You might be eating some foods for the first time, or at least in a greater quantity than before.

You may experience rumbling in your stomach, and you may also find you are a bit more gassy and going to the restroom more frequently. These are all signs that your body is learning how to process and digest the new food you are giving it, while at the same time, eliminating toxins. (I'm trying to be polite, but I'm talking about poop. This is the best and most immediate way for your body to get the bad stuff out.)

During the early part of the diet, and especially during the cleanse, you may experience headaches and even mild flu-like symptoms. This is sometimes referred to as "carbohydrate flu," which happens when you dramatically reduce your processed food intake, which you MUST do to reverse and heal your fatty liver.

Your emotional state may be a little wishy-washy when you start. Dizziness and physical weakness, moodiness and fatigue, low energy and constant trips to the bathroom are *very common*.

However, over time (usually a short time), you will gain newfound clarity. For many people, they discover their true purpose in life after a cleanse. That certainly happened to me. In fact, you could say my fatty liver was **directly** responsible for the total health transformation that I'm still living. ;-)

Keys To Feeling Good

The biggest piece of advice I can give you is to remember to drink plenty of liquids, especially during the cleanse. You will be moving so much junk out of your body, your waste might have a higher water content than it normally does (and it may smell particularly bad).

Keep a water bottle or glass handy throughout the day, sipping and refilling it constantly. Stay hydrated at all times.

You may also be eating more food than you are used to. While fasting has its place, this program is **not** about fasting or keto or paleo or anything like that. It's about **stopping the hurt** and **feeding the liver** healthy foods that help it rebuild itself and nourish your body at the same time.

Smaller, More Frequent Meals

During the cleanse, it is better to eat 6 or 7 small snacks throughout the day than to try to stuff yourself during mealtimes. This makes the elimination process easier on your liver and the rest of your digestive system.

To ensure you are getting all the healthy protein you need, make sure you're eating plenty of nuts, sprouts, and leafy greens. You should also be enjoying beans and legumes when you are eating normally.

BONUS

Fatty Liver Friendly Recipes

Here are a couple of simple recipes to get you started. Aim for easy and quick, and remember to focus on the whole-food plant-based approach as opposed to eating meats and dairy.

Simple Salad

An easy way to get a diverse amount of liver-healing foods into your body is to make a salad once a day. Purchase an extra large salad bowl, one that you would use to serve your entire family.

Slice, dice, chop, shave and grate your favorite vegetables on the healthy liver shopping list. Store the container in your fridge without dressing the salad. Make one of these large salads in the morning, and you can munch on it all day long. Instead of slathering it with unhealthy dressing, use extra-virgin olive oil and red-wine vinegar, or use the simple and healthy salad dressing recipe below.

Simple Salad Dressing

This is my standard salad dressing, light, easy, and tasty.

Ingredients

2 tablespoons of extra virgin olive or walnut oil
2 tablespoon of apple cider or red wine vinegar
1 tablespoon of dijon mustard
Juice from 1/2 lemon
Salt and pepper to taste

Instructions

Add to small container, shake vigorously, pour on salad when ready to eat.

Simple Stirfry

Another easy way to get your vegetables is with a stirfry, which is both easy and healthy. I like to pour mine over brown rice, or even better, quinoa for a high-protein and filling meal. Add any veggies you have in your fridge since this is a great way to use up extra food you may have around.

Ingredients

2 tablespoons extra virgin olive oil

2 cloves garlic, chopped

1 finger (2") of turmeric, chopped

1 finger (2") of ginger, chopped

1/2 green bell pepper, chopped

1/2 red bell pepper, chopped

1 small zucchini, chopped

1 cup broccoli, chopped

1 cup carrots, chopped

1/2 cup green or yellow string beans, chopped

1/2 cup red or golden beets, diced

1/2 cup shiitake mushrooms, chopped

1/2 cup kale or chard, chopped

Instructions

Stir fry in a large pan or wok, serve over brown rice or quinoa.

Gourmet Spanish Gazpacho

This is an incredibly easy, super healthy cold soup you can make, and then stick in the fridge to enjoy for a few days. You can peel your tomatoes and roast the red pepper first, or just throw them in the blender, and voila, you have a delicious, gourmet soup that's healthy, raw, and full of life.

Ingredients

2 lbs, of tomatoes (seeded)

1 large peeled cucumber

1 medium red pepper (seeded)

3 - 5 garlic cloves

1/4 cup of extra virgin olive oil

Salt and pepper to taste.

Instructions

Mix in a blender, food processor, or Vita-mix and refrigerate. Lasts 3 - 5 days.

Golden Milk

This is a delicious beverage that has the power to reduce joint pain and inflammation over your entire body. Basically, you mix turmeric and black pepper with a heated nut milk (like coconut or almond). Many health-food stores have pre-packaged golden milk mixes, but it's easy enough to create your own. If you take blood-thinning medications, consult your physician before taking curcumin or turmeric as a daily supplement since there can be unintended interactions.

Ingredients

1 tablespoon of freshly ground or 1/2 tablespoon dried turmeric
1/2 tablespoon of freshly ground black pepper
2 cups fresh filtered water
2 cups coconut or almond milk

Instructions

Mix turmeric, pepper, and water in a pan. Bring to a boil, cover and let sit for 15 minutes. Strain and mix liquid with coconut or almond milk. You may make a large batch and refrigerate. Lasts about a week.

Veggie Chili

This is a very flexible recipe, and like the stirfry, you can use what you want, or delete ingredients you don't. I like to make veggie chili when I have a lot of random leftover veggies in my fridge from other recipes that need to be used up.

Ingredients

2 tablespoons extra virgin olive oil
1/3 onion, rough chopped
2 bay leaves
1 tablespoon ground cumin
2 tablespoons dried oregano
1 tablespoon salt
3 cloves garlic, chopped
1 jalapeño pepper, seeded and chopped
3 tablespoons chili powder
1 tablespoon ground black pepper
3 stalks celery, chopped
1 medium zucchini, chopped

2 green or red bell peppers, chopped

2 small cans chopped green chiles

3 cans (28-ounce) whole peeled tomatoes, drained and chopped

1 can kidney beans, drained

1 can garbanzo beans, drained

1 can black beans, drained

Instructions

Add oil, onion, and spices to pan and cook until onions are translucent. Then add all other ingredients to a large pot, and simmer on stove for 60 - 90 minutes as everything cooks together. You can also make this in a slow-cooker or crock pot. Serve in a bowl, or over brown rice.

Avocado Flatbread Toast

This is my healthy take on avocado toast, minus the bread. It's a delicious snack, or you can double it and turn it into a meal or side dish.

Ingredients

1 medium avocado

1/2 lemon or lime, juiced

Salt and pepper to taste

1 tsp. of sesame seeds (optional)

Sprouted corn tortillas or rice crackers

Instructions

Smash ingredients in a bowl, scoop and spread on tortilla or cracker.

CONCLUSION

You Are My Inspiration

Congratulations are in order. You have taken health and well-being into your own hands. That is a powerfully liberating feeling, something nobody can take away from you. I can't tell you how honored and inspired I am to have you as part of the **Fix Your Fatty Liver** program.

Now it is decision time...

Are you going to adopt some new dietary practices, pay attention to what you put in your body, and move towards a plant-based diet as part of your new life?

Are you willing to finally start a daily walk, move your body, and maybe even join that gym?

Are you going to seek out positive people, and start avoiding situations that add drama, stress, and toxicity to your day?

It is entirely up to you. Perhaps you'll start slowly, and see for yourself how you feel as you implement each new step. Or maybe you are ready for a breakthrough change that has the power to transform your life forever, and intend to implement this program completely.

I believe you are going to feel so good after going through this material, you'll want to stay that way all the time. That's what happened to me: I look and feel so incredibly healthy, why would I ever go back?

I really hope you consider doing the same. The benefits are undeniable and significant, and not only can this help you live longer, but it can also improve your quality of life for the years you still have.

Make a healthy promise to yourself

Try eating all of the wonderfully nutritious and delicious foods in the Fatty Liver Diet for a few months. Give the cleanse a shot. Eliminate negative influences in your life, and become familiar with loving and respecting your body.

Try some of the daily affirmations to start your morning, and turn your bad habits into good ones. Over time the constant repetition of your affirmations and new healthy habits will create a powerful mindset that promotes positivity, reduce stress and anxiety, and create a continued desire to remain healthy.

Remember that your environment plays a huge part in influencing your behavior. It may be tough, and you might even have to search out new friends that embrace your healthy attitude, but it's worth it.

You may have to change your physical environment as well, which could be as easy as decluttering your home of toxins and distractions, or as hard as moving from where you currently live. But now you know–something needs to be done.

All of us at the Fix Your Fatty Liver program hope this is only the beginning for you on your path to incredible health and wellness. We join everyone who made this program possible (and there were dozens) in wishing you the best moving forward.

Regards,

Jonathan Mizel
Creator, Fix Your Fatty Liver

Resources and References

- Our Fatty Liver Facebook Group

https://www.facebook.com/FattyLiverProtocol/

- Your free book on Emotional Eating by Glenn Livingston

http://fattyliverbook.com/emotional-eating

- Tips on starting a mindfulness program

https://www.mindful.org

- Check the glycemic index of your foods

http://www.glycemicindex.com/

- The juicer I use

http://www.target.com/p/omega-8006-low-speed-masticating-juicer/

- Sold to the Highest Bidder – the Fatally Flawed Food Pyramid

https://www.earlytorise.com/our-no-hassle-plan-for-healthy-living/sold-to-the-highest-bidder-the-fatally-flawed-food-pyramid/

- 50 Years Ago, Sugar Industry Quietly Paid Scientists To Point Blame At Fat

https://www.npr.org/sections/thetwo-way/2016/09/13/493739074/50-years-ago-sugar-industry-quietly-paid-scientists-to-point-blame-at-fat

- How Candy Makers Shape Science

https://apnews.com/f9483d554430445fa6566bb0aaa293d1

- How Much Do Doctors Learn About Nutrition?

https://health.usnews.com/wellness/food/articles/2016-12-07/how-much-do-doctors-learn-about-nutrition

- Body's response to repetitive laughter is similar to the effect of repetitive exercise, study finds

https://www.sciencedaily.com/releases/2010/04/100426113058.htm

- Science proves the positive power of morning rituals

https://www.inspiringleadershipnow.com/the-power-of-the-early-morning-ritual-why-science-believes-it-makes-for-a-high-achieving-leader/

- Explaining a parasympathetic state

https://adrenalfatiguesolution.com/fight-or-flight-vs-rest-and-digest/

- What happens to your body when you eat sugar

https://www.self.com/story/this-is-exactly-what-happens-to-your-body-when-you-eat-a-ton-of-sugar

- Dangers of Glyphosate

https://www.nature.com/articles/srep39328

- Kaiser Whole Food Plant Based diet booklet

https://share.kaiserpermanente.org/wp-content/uploads/2015/10/The-Plant-Based-Diet-booklet.pdf

- Unhealthy effect of sunscreen on your liver

http://www.mnn.com/health/fitness-well-being/blogs/why-i-dont-wear-sunscreen

- Dangers of Acetaminophen

https://craighospital.org/uploads/Educational-PDFs/717.Acetaminophen-and-Liver-Damage-FDA.pdf

- Eat Right: The Benefits Of Beets For Triathletes

http://www.triathlete.com/2015/02/nutrition/eat-right-the-benefits-of-beets_89673

- Probiotics Restore Bowel Flora and Improve Liver Enzymes in Human Alcohol-Induced Liver Injury: A Pilot Study

https://www.ncbi.nlm.nih.gov/pmc/articles/PMC2630703/

- Does Vitamin B Regenerate the Liver?

http://healthyeating.sfgate.com/vitamin-b-regenerate-liver-4602.html

- Fifteen ways to love your liver

http://www.doctoryourself.com/liver_15_ways.html

- Hepatoprotective effect of Rhodiola imbricata rhizome against paracetamol-induced liver toxicity in rats https://www.ncbi.nlm.nih.gov/pmc/articles/PMC4191600/

- Blood pH considerations

http://www.medicinenet.com/script/main/art.asp?articlekey=10001

- University of California Glyphosate study

https://detoxproject.org/1321-2/

- Benefits of Oatmeal for Fatty Liver Disease

https://nutritionfacts.org/2017/02/09/benefits-of-oatmeal-for-fatty-liver-disease/

- Walnuts and Diabetes

https://www.ncbi.nlm.nih.gov/pubmed/15983525

- Glycemic Index

https://www.webmd.com/diabetes/guide/glycemic-index-good-versus-bad-carbs

- Benefits of broccoli

https://nutritionfacts.org/2013/07/18/broccoli-boosts-liver-detox-enzymes/

- Benefits of sulforaphane

https://www.sciencedaily.com/releases/2017/03/170307100402.htm

- Insecticides and liver health

http://www.hepatitiscentral.com/news/mosquito_repell/

- Sugar vs. Cocaine

abc13.com/health/study-sugar-is-as-addictive-as-cocaine/533979/

- Probiotics and gut health: A special focus on liver diseases

https://www.ncbi.nlm.nih.gov/pmc/articles/PMC2811790/

- List of unhealthy hair dyes and healthy alternatives

http://www.greathealthnaturally.co.uk/2013/07/25/is-your-hair-dye-causing-a-progressive-fatal-liver-disease/

- Beet Kvass recipe

https://wellnessmama.com/9087/beet-kvass-recipe/

- Breathing exercises

https://www.drweil.com/health-wellness/body-mind-spirit/stress-anxiety/breathing-three-exercises/

- Turmeric/curcumin supplement

http://TumericExtract.org

NOTES:

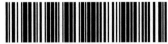

Made in the USA
Columbia, SC
22 April 2018